THE BUDDY SYSTEM DIET

Lisa Carruthers MS RD

Copyright © 2013 Lisa Carruthers MS RD

All rights reserved.

ISBN: 1475036574

ISBN 13: 9781475036572

Library of Congress Control Number: 2012905300
CreateSpace, North Charleston, SC

DEDICATION

This book is dedicated to Benny Cuckier who continues to make me laugh.

TABLE OF CONTENTS

Foreword		vii
Acknowledgements		ix
Introduction		xi
1.	*Getting Started*	1
2.	*Goals*	5
3.	*What is The Buddy System?*	9
4.	*Food Journaling*	13
5.	*Progress*	23
6.	*Motivation to Keep You Going*	27
7.	*Additional Nutrition Tips*	33
8.	*Move It Like Jagger*	41
9.	*Meal Plans*	45
10.	*Recipes*	61
11.	*References*	119

FOREWARD

Food journaling is one of the most powerful tools for weight loss. The idea behind this book is too teach people how to be successful with journaling. We hear about writing down what we eat, but there are some important concepts that aren't often taught. For instance portion size and method of cooking.

Accountability is another key tool for maintaining weight loss progress. It's important to have someone to check in with whether it's a Registered Dietitian, an athletic trainer, or your friend.

I talk about how important motivators are later in the book. I am just another motivator with a different style of presenting the same information. Eventhough most people intuitively know which foods are healthy, and which foods are high in calories; it often takes just the right voice for those realities to sink in.

Brevity is another difference here. You will see I like to get to the point. There are many in-depth nutrition or diet books on the market, and I believe many people like to get to the bottom line. If you are like me and see a book that is bigger than the Yellow Pages, you might feel discouraged before you even start reading.

Also, my intention is to use the principles in this book in conjunction with any other weight loss plan of choice. I also provide meal plans and recipes that can be used for weight loss too.

> I commend you for *thinking* about weight loss and the process that is involved. The next step is ***action***.

ACKNOWLEDGEMENT

My thanks to my mother, Deanna Lazear, for her tireless review of recipes and continued support. I would also like to thank Stan Fridstein for his encouragement and introducing me to Createspace. And many thanks to Ron Ogulnick for providing me with a quiet and stress-free environment to work.

INTRODUCTION

The primary reason I decided to write this book was so my clients would have a reference tool to use in conjunction with their nutrition counseling sessions. I always hated to see my clients writing copious notes during our sessions and struggling to capture every word that I said. I finally realized that it would be more efficient to provide my clients with the same information but as a handout or book. The printed material would be available for them to review later. That would leave us with more focused communication during the sessions.

It took me awhile to put these few pages together. I was always afraid of inadvertently copying what another author had written but the reality is that there aren't really any new ways to lose weight. Basically it still falls back to the straightforward yet elusive formula of calories in versus calories out.

I believe the primary difference between my book and the millions of other weight loss books on the market is that this is my voice. I present a different style or a unique way of saying the same things you may have heard before.

I hope this book will help any of you who have chosen to read it. Weight loss is challenging and can be frustrating.

We live in a society that promotes unhealthy behaviors and offers little support.

We have to work harder to overcome the obstacles presented in our daily lives. Hopefully this book will assist you in meeting that challenge.

CHAPTER ONE

GETTING STARTED

The first step in a journey to lose weight is a difficult endeavor. This initial phase is just acknowledging that it's time to make a change. I don't know if it's *the* most difficult part of your journey, because there are many bumps in the road. Actually, there may be haystacks and sinkholes along the way. There will be moments when it seems like you are the only one on the planet who can't lose weight. You might feel as if your DNA is flawed. You might feel cursed. You might feel like everyone knows something that you don't. There will be times when you want to stop trying because it's too much work for such slow results. Perhaps you've gone to your doctor because you are positive there is a problem with your thyroid. You might be thinking, "Bob down the street looks fabulous, why didn't I have the same results on the same diet plan?" Sometimes you just get tired of talking and thinking about food.

The reality is that it really can be difficult to lose weight. It is a commitment. It is effort. It is planning and preparation. It's picking yourself up, and dusting yourself off when you eat that entire chocolate cake and stop exercising for a week because of it. Plain and simple, it's hard work. But, if you think about it, anything in life that is worth having takes effort.

You don't wake up in the morning with a college degree, a paycheck, or a painted masterpiece, for example. Whatever was important to you, was planned for.

You prepared. You made arrangements. It took time. Always remember; *planning and preparation are key* factors for weight loss success.

One of my clients, *Benny*, weighed about 500 pounds when I first met him. He has now lost over 200 pounds. The inspiring part of his weight loss was that he did it with diet and exercise only. He didn't have surgery or take any type of weight loss medication or supplements. On the first day of our journey together he said, "I feel like I'm at the bottom of Mount Everest looking up". My response was, "Yes, you are". He had been told in the past that it would just take a little willpower to lose the weight. Personally, I think that advice was flawed because it ignores the plain fact that lasting weight loss is a process. That process is rarely a linear decline down. There are also typically weight plateaus along the way that can last for a month or more. Habits and behaviors need to change for solid weight loss to occur. Benny could always muster up enough "willpower" to follow a diet, but when the diet was over he didn't have a clue what to do next. Will power is about *not* eating a particular food at a particular moment, which is important. However, will power doesn't address the gradual changes that need to occur in your life so that you can be happy and content with the food you are consuming.

Don't let anyone fool you. There is no magic bullet for healthy, long-term weight loss. It's True Grit and effort, and hopefully the fact that you are here right now reading this means that an internal switch has been turned on. You have decided. You are ready.

You *will* be successful. Just by deciding that now is the time to start, is a momentous move in the right direction. You can't have one foot in the door and one foot out.

You need to walk in all the way and shut the door behind you. In other words, you can't be indecisive about the decision to start making a change. It's either yes or no.

After reading that last paragraph and doing some real soul searching you may realize that you're not one hundred percent in. That's okay. Don't try half-hearted today because you might likely fail and re-affirm what you already thought about yourself, *"I can't lose weight."* I'm not telling you to forget about it altogether though. You know if you need to lose weight, and you know if your health warrants weight loss. Set a start date and write it on a calendar somewhere. Maybe it will be next week, or perhaps in two weeks. Prepare yourself mentally to begin, but don't wait too long.

Hopefully the information laid out here will be helpful for you. Don't think of it as your last chance for successful weight loss. What works for one person, may not work for another. Also, don't think that just because you are reading this, that the weight will magically fall off. You are the magic. You are the one that makes it all happen. This information should be used as a motivator and for sound advice. If it doesn't motivate you, then please try something else. Don't give up. We are all motivated by different things and different people.

There are also many things around us that can diminish our motivation. I think a big de-motivator for many people is that we are lured into thinking we should be something that we are not. For starters, the media tells us we should look a certain way, even though the people in print, television, or movies may not even look that way in person either. It's amazing what computers, make-up and lighting can do. Take a look at The Dove® Campaign for Real Beauty.com. There you will see just how fake some of these images are that we compare ourselves to.

The other standard that is difficult to live up to is preparing gourmet meals every day. The television chefs and magazines entice us into thinking we need to make every dish a work of art and a gastronomical feast. It all becomes overwhelming if you don't know how to boil water and you have 15 minutes to prepare dinner. People often feel so much pressure that they just give up. This is when we get in the car and drive through a fast food restaurant. A few years ago my mother healthfully lost 25 pounds, and I assumed it was from the years of solicited advice I had given her. She admitted that she lost the weight after reading a popular and nutritionally sound diet book written by a media physician. I was a little incensed, but she explained that the book actually reinforced what I had told her, and it was just a new resource for motivation. I then realized that it didn't matter the source of her motivation, because she still lost the weight by eating right and exercising. Soon after that, I proceeded to begin my own book!

Try to think about going back to the basics and keeping things simple, simple, simple. Be more concerned with the nutritional content rather than how it looks or tastes. I know that may seem contrary to what others say. I know you eat with your eyes first and it should taste delicious. But I believe that we have become out of balance with what we expect from our food. I remember when going to a local coffee shop was considered a treat. Now we go to restaurants where we admire the culinary artistry or we enjoy the complicated layers of infused flavors. Food has become our primary source of entertainment. Even fast food has become "gourmet." Simple ingredients and basic recipes are all you need. Savor the gourmet for special occasions.

One last thought, if you feel like you're at the bottom of Mount Everest or that it will take a miracle to lose the weight, then start taking those baby steps or create that miracle yourself. Don't wait any longer. Make it happen!

CHAPTER TWO

GOAL

Now that you've made the commitment to lose weight, it's time to make a plan. Remember *planning and preparation*.

The first part of your plan is to determine approximately how much weight you are going to lose. I recommend starting with small increments of weight. For example, start with a goal of losing maybe five or ten pounds When you achieve that goal, then commit to losing another five or ten pounds and so on until you've reached the peak of your personal Mount Everest.

Many professionals refer to various "tables" to determine if a patient or client is overweight. I believe that you already know if you're overweight, and that you don't really need a chart or table to tell you so. However, the tables can be useful in helping you establish the weight range to determine your risk factors for morbidity and mortality. Sometimes people become overly focused on a pre-determined ideal weight that it's psychologically counterproductive. The prescribed weight goal from a table may seem so over-whelming and impossible to achieve that the person gives up before trying. This is why it's helpful to break up your ultimate weight goal into successive mini goals.

So, let's look briefly at what some of those tables or guides mean anyway.

The pediatric growth charts are used by pediatricians to track the height and weight of children as they grow and mature.

These charts also monitor the body mass index (BMI)-for-age of a child. They are useful tools for tracking the weight progress of a child and obviously not used for adults. In turn, adult charts should not be used for children. The growth charts for both medical professionals and the public can be found at The Centers for Disease Control (CDC) website at www.cdc.gov/growthcharts/.

The Metropolitan Height and Weight charts were some of the original weight charts and were developed by the insurance companies in 1943. They were initially used to determine a persons' mortality risk based on height, weight, and frame size. Later on they were used to determine if an adult man or woman was overweight.

Next came along *Broca's* Index. This is a quick method of calculating Ideal Body Weight (IBW) for men and women. For women, start with one hundred pounds for the first five feet, then add five pounds for each additional inch of height. So according to this method, the ideal body weight for a five foot three inch woman would be 115 pounds. For men its 110 pounds for the first five feet, then five pounds for every inch after that. This method doesn't account for age, muscle mass, or frame size.

Today the BMI is considered the best tool for determining overweight and morbid obesity in adults.

I feel this is a good measurement to determine trends in large groups of people and ideal weight ranges for individuals, but it doesn't address the individual's muscle mass. Still, BMI can be helpful in determining an appropriate weight *range* for someone.

I think the best way to determine your final and short-term weight goals is by using more than one method of IBW indicators or weight measurements. There are convenient BMI calculators, as discussed previously, to help determine your appropriate weight range. This easy to use calculator can be found at the National Institute of Healths' website www.nhlbisupport.com/bmi/.

Another good tool to include is waist measurement. The greater your waist size, the increased chance of developing heart disease or diabetes. Men should have a waist circumference of forty inches or below. A woman's waist circumference should be thirty-five inches or less. Check this by placing a soft tape measure around your waist and rest it about one inch above your hip bones.

Now, think back ten years ago. What was your weight then and how has it changed over the years? Has there been a slow and steady gain of just a few pounds per year? Or was there a sudden increase in weight due to a life changing event? Looking back now, what do you think was an appropriate weight for *you*? When you were at this "ideal" weight did you have energy? Were you eating healthy food? Were you exercising? Now ask yourself, is that weight realistic to maintain in a healthy way today? Was this before kids, family obligations, work responsibilities, etc? Were you a single man or woman going to the gym every night after work because that was your social outlet? Were you eating a bowl of cereal every night for dinner because it was simple? Did you have alcohol once a month socially because there was no one to share a good bottle of wine with on occasion? Are you now taking a medication that affects your weight? Did you have an injury that changed the type or intensity of your exercise? Is this former weight realistic to maintain now within all the constraints that life has to offer now. Also, consider maintaining this realistic weight in a healthier way than ever before. Lets' put all of this information together and come up with a weight range that works for you. Use the BMI to determine your weight range goal. Remember this ideal weight range might be different than what it was ten years ago. Use the waist circumference measurement to help see real-time changes.

Changes in clothing size will work in the same way. The scale is useful in monitoring long-term changes. It will also keep you on track and accountable on a daily basis. Unfortunately it can easily fluctuate with fluid changes. Meaning, it may read an artificially higher weight and cause you some discouragement. Finally, think about the lifestyle you will be happy maintaining.

*Now that you've determined your long term goal for weight loss, write it down and forget about it. Keep in mind that number may change as you re-evaluate your goals during the weight loss process. As you lose weight you may decide at a certain point that you've lost enough, and that maintenance is realistic to maintain this new weight or body size. Just remember that weight is a number on a scale and can be influenced by many factors. Don't be stuck on that number which is your long-term goal. Instead focus on short term goals. Losing five pounds at a time is a realistic goal to start with. Although the objective doesn't have to be measured in pounds. You may want to focus on inches around the waist, or even clothing size. I like to use several measurements of some sort incase the scale is lying that day. Remember Benny looking up the mountain?

He had to start with one step at a time. The same is for you. Allow yourself many small successes along the way, instead of just one big reward at the end. Why not feel good about yourself and your accomplishments now, not just a year from now? The small successes now will give you the confidence to continue when the going gets tough and you're ready to throw in the towel. Some weeks you may not see any progress at all. Hang in there another week or two and you will.

If you are currently a man or woman over the age of about thirty, it's easy to compare now with a time in your life when you wanted to fit into a certain tight skirt or pair of jeans. All it took was "starving" for a few days and then the weight was gone. Not only was that an unhealthy way to lose the extra weight; that quick weight loss method will never happen again. Primarily because you are older now and your environment has changed. Metabolism changes over time and tends to slow down rather than increase. It's important to accept who you are now and how your body responds to weight loss currently, otherwise you may become very disappointed.

If you are younger than 30 years old, it's important to focus on slow steady weight loss. You want to avoid a life of yo-yo dieting, and you want to develop lifelong healthy habits.

Having said all that, just know you have to work harder the older you get. Don't become complacent. The benefits will be beyond what you expect. So think about your goal and/or goals and write them down on paper and sign your name to it. This will be a commitment you are making to yourself.

CHAPTER THREE

WHAT IS THE BUDDY SYSTEM?

Throughout life most people need support from others to help us accomplish our life's ambitions and aspirations. This may be in the form of encouragement to accomplish a lofty goal. The support may simply be to provide acknowledgement and companionship as we live through the pleasures and heartaches of each day. I believe the majority of us also need support from others to lose weight, but we don't necessarily recognize that. Sometimes, we can be a little stubborn at times and try to do *everything* alone.

Often people will say that they gained the weight themselves and they should be able to lose it without help. Even though I am a Registered Dietitian, I need support to stay on track with my diet, exercise, and weight maintenance. My family supports my efforts to eat healthy and exercise. My best friends are Registered Dietitians and personal trainers. I regularly hike with friends (The Heartbreak Hiking Fools). My personal physician provides encouragement when we discuss my health goals. I take group classes like cycling or yoga at the gym. I read health and nutrition articles. I watch television programs related to health. I also use various tracking systems for recording my food intake and activity expenditure. I am constantly utilizing the support systems and motivators I have around me. And, quite frankly the fact that I spend my entire day counseling people for weight loss keeps me motivated as well!

AH HA! Here is a key component to successful, consistent, and lasting weight loss. It is **accountability**.

Think about this for a minute. Why is the diet "business" a billion dollar industry? For one thing there are a lot of people trying to lose weight. But more importantly, we are always trying to find that one perfect *motivator*.

We search for someone or something that will propel us into doing what we know needs to be done. We look for that magical program that will make weight loss materialize without much effort. But then when we feel a particular program isn't "perfect" and our weight loss goals aren't accomplished, we move on to another program or plan.

There are a "million" weight loss programs and plans out there, but the bottom line will always be less calorie in and more physical movement.

You all know this but still hold out and hope for something different or hope that somehow the work will be done for you because it's difficult to change habits. It's also difficult to be consistent and patient.

The overall process to losing weight is not a mystery, but the tricky part is sticking with it. One of the things that we are looking for in all those "diets" is the accountability and the cheerleader. We want to be prodded and praised when we'd rather stop trying so hard. We want someone to say, "Good for you"! after we've passed up the dessert. Ultimately, there are two (among other) important factors for successful weight loss. These are *accountability* and *motivation*. These two valuable ingredients for healthy weight loss can be combined with any reasonable diet plan for sustained success.

Is this book another gimmick? Well, yes it is. There's nothing different about the "bones" of this plan. It's just another approach that hopefully will work for a few more people. There are so many different weight loss strategies available now and as you've heard "no one diet fits all". This is just another presentation and tool based on a healthy lifestyle.

You can use this plan alone or pair it with another "diet" if you like. Think of this as an opportunity to customize your own program. Make it a plan that finally works for the individual that you are. Remember this is all your own effort, but without having to do it alone. In other words, you must be an active participant in your own weight loss while using the tool of accountability.

So here it is. You need support, motivation, and effort. The effort already started with you, you opened this book and started to read. Now you need that little "kick in the pants" to keep you motivated to continue on. This is where another person comes in handy. This is your weight loss "buddy." Your buddy will provide the accountability and motivation or support. You will also do the same for your buddy, which in turn will increase your motivation.

What Is The Buddy System?

The premise of this plan and name of the book is to find someone to be accountable to and who will motivate you. You in turn, will provide the same support back. The *magic* actually happens when someone is accountable to you. It's similar to the way a doctor becomes proficient. During medical school the intern is instructed to "learn one, do one, teach one." You can become proficient at your own weight loss or maintenance by helping or *teaching* someone else.

How do you pick your buddy? First think of someone that is able to provide the same time commitment as you. Look around within your own family. Look around at work.

Maybe there's someone in your neighborhood or religious institution. Your buddy doesn't have to be someone that you know very well.

This person could be a relative or friend out of state. The communicating can be done on the telephone or on the computer. You might even ask your physician to put the word out to other patients that need to lose weight. You don't need a partner with the same exact goals as you. Maybe you want to lose five pounds and your buddy wants to lose five inches. You can even follow another meal plan or program other than what is provided in this book. Now, if you are one of my clients reading this I realize it's a one-sided relationship, but similar principles still apply.

In this book I provide you with a "Reader's Digest" version of nutrition tips and education. It's some basics to get you started and to clear up some confusing information you may have picked up previously. There is a list of nutrition references in the back if you would like a reputable resource for further information.

I give you tips along the way. Most are from my clients and friends who have had brilliant ideas about food and weight loss. So much of what works is by trial and error and it's great to pass those insights on to others.

I provided you with meal plans and recipes to help you along the way. As I explained earlier, you may find another healthy plan that suits your preferences or lifestyle better than mine. Please use whatever appeals to you.

I have provided three calorie levels of plans 1200, 1500, and 1800. All of the recipes included have calories listed on the bottom of each page so you'll know how to fit them into your plan. Lastly, I provided you with some structure to use with your buddy. Yes, this includes the dreaded food journal! The journal is a key component to this plan, and the results are unbelievably beneficial.

I realize that many people find the idea of journaling very tedious and time-consuming, but there are so many ways to journal that can be time-efficient. Once you see the results you'll be hooked for life.

Now, go find your buddy and I'll see you on the next page!

CHAPTER FOUR

FOOD JOURNALING

It's simple and somewhat tedious but food journaling is one of the most successful tools in the challenge of weight loss. First of all, what is food journaling?

A food journal is simply a diary of what you eat during the day. The most basic way to journal is to take a piece of paper, a notebook, a document page on your computer, or notes on a smart phone and write down what you eat during the day. There are also great computer programs and smart phone apps that are designed just for this reason. You can record your food consumption as you go throughout the day or wait until the evening and write everything down then. This means everything!

For the journaling to be effective, you should write down every single bite of food you eat. This includes the lick of peanut butter off the knife after you've made your kids' lunch. It includes standing with the refrigerator door open and popping a bite here and a bite there into your mouth. It's the cake batter off the spoon and bowl after the cake is already is in the oven. Also, it might be a few French fries off your friend's plate in that restaurant. It might be a few sips from your spouses' drink. I could go on, but you all know exactly what I mean.

Each little bite here and there could potentially add up to hundreds of extra unwanted calories. You can see already that you might avoid eating extra calories because of the hassle of having to write it all down!

I believe we think that all those extra calories don't really count. We tend to forget about those "bites" because they didn't seem significant in the first place. The reality is that all those little bites here and there could potentially add up to several pounds of unwanted weight over the course of a year.

A simple "bite" can easily be 50 calories. A handful of nuts can be up to 200 calories. These calories really add up over the course of a day, and the drawback is that you don't even feel like you've eaten anything.

It's not like you had a conscious snack or meal and feel satisfied. Food journaling helps us bring those calories in the forefront. No more denial. They're there in black and white. You're thinking about it now. There's nowhere to hide.

Here's more of the magic of journaling; when you are in the habit of writing everything you eat, you often notice some habits that you may not have even been conscious of. Are you hitting the vending machine at work at a certain time every day? Do you drink extra calories of juice or milk straight from the carton without thinking about it? What about grabbing a cookie in the lunchroom at work? Maybe it's a piece or two of chocolate in your accountant's office. Or do you finish the food off your kids' plate before doing the dishes?

The other important thing is that the journal shows you what you are doing that's positive.

Now your buddy can look and say, 'wow, you really eat a lot of vegetables". Or maybe they can say, "You've really decreased those cooking fats'. Not only do you have the journal to keep *you* honest, you now have another pair of eyes looking at what you are doing.

Just think how proud you'll feel when your partner sees that you eat bran flakes with blueberries and skim milk for breakfast, instead of chocolate cake washed down with cola. (You know this happens).

It sounds a little corny, but this is positive reinforcement and we all need it. No matter what the praise is, we all respond to it. We are then more likely to repeat the behaviors. The food diary helps you to take down the veil of secrecy. Having another person look at it helps you to be accountable. Even if you are "artificially" changing behaviors because someone will be looking at what you are doing, it doesn't matter. You are still changing behaviors. Those changes in behavior will eventually become habit. You might also have some indiscretions or less than proud moments during the week as well. It's your partner's job to point out areas for possible change. Without the diary, golden opportunities for change might never occur.

Some of you might be thinking that this is just a crutch or a trick. I say so what. If it helps you to get into habits that you can sustain, I am all for it! You can look back at a previous weeks' journal and you might be surprised at what you see. Whatever denial you might have will be there in black and white. It's much easier to fix what you know is wrong rather than just thinking that you can't lose weight for some unknown reason.

Here is an interesting thing to do before you start your regular journaling. Let's say it's the day or so before you actually start with dietary and lifestyle changes. Write everything down. Let everything hang out, so to speak. Take that piece of paper with your recorded food on it and put it away. Look at it several months later, and you will be shocked at what you see. Now, you can share it with your buddy. Sometimes we don't really notice the small gradual changes until some length of time has passed. This is a golden opportunity for more positive reinforcement.

WHAT TO RECORD IN YOUR JOURNAL

I have included pages at the end of the book for you to copy for your journal pages. You can also write or purchase your own diary. Remember it should be legible enough for your partner to read it. If you have poor penmanship, I would suggest recording your diary on the computer or as a text on your mobile phone. Another option would be to use one of the many food diaries available online. Many of these are free, and they will add up calories for you as well. If you use one of these programs, simply exchange passwords with your buddy. The use of the computer would be essential if you will not be meeting your buddy in person, whether you e-mail your diary as an attached document or subscribe to a program. See references for some of the on-line diet programs available. Record the time of day when you eat. This is important for catching some binges. If the first time you eat all day is 5:00 PM and you've consumed enough food for a family of four, then it will be easy for your partner **and you** to see what went wrong that day.

Obviously you want to record what you have eaten, but just as important, document the ***portion size***. Be consistent with the recorded portions and try not to list "a bite", or "a handful" Record your foods as household measurements that you are both familiar with. If you say "teaspoon", think of a measuring teaspoon and not the spoon you use to eat cereal with. If you say a cup, then refer to a measuring cup not a juice glass or a coffee mug.

Add a hunger scale to the time when you have eaten. I like to use one through five. One is "starving" and "five" is stuffed. This hunger scale helps you to identify if you are mindlessly eating, or if you've gone too long without eating.

Lastly, record your physical activity. Notice I didn't say "exercise." All movement counts, so record it. If you took a flight of stairs, or walked through the local mall shopping, record it. Beside the activity, list the amount of time actually doing the activity. Of course, if you went to the gym then record the amount of time doing cardio, stretching, or resistance as well.

The overall goal of the food and activity diary is to receive and provide positive feedback while identifying areas for change. Do not expect perfection from yourself or your partner. Changing habits takes time and is a process. The following list can help you look for specifics in the journals. Don't expect to fulfill everything on the list everyday or even every week. It is simply a quick and easy check-list of dietary goals to work towards. Although you need to record in your journal daily, you can be flexible with your partner as to when you review them. I would suggest a weekly review, but you can review them every other week as well. Whatever is convenient for you and your partner.

HOW TO REVIEW YOUR BUDDY'S JOURNAL

The most important thing to remember here is to accentuate the positive!!! Remember, you are the cheerleader. Carefully read what your partner has written. Look at each food. Look at the entire day. What can you say positive about this day. Did your partner eat fruit? Did they eat vegetables? How about some whole grains, or legumes? How little or what kind of fat did they eat? What about exercise? How many days was breakfast eaten? Find the positives and congratulate them. Remember, your partner is probably berating themselves for the way they've eaten this week, so it's your job to pull him/her out of that. After you've reviewed the week and made as many positive comments as possible, go back and provide some constructive criticism. Remember that no one is harder on us than ourselves so don't be brutal here. Just pick 1 or 2 things you see as the most significant ways they can improve for the next week. For example; could they have eaten more fruit? Could they have done a little more exercise? What about salad dressing, could they switch to low fat instead of fully loaded? Maybe you know of a brand of dressing you like that you could share.

This tool is meant as a helping aid for both of you. Don't be punitive or a taskmaster. Losing weight is difficult and you are there to keep your partner feeling positive when the going gets tough. Also, try to keep the focus on being healthy and not about being "skinny". Improved health is really the overall prize anyway. For example, give praise for using olive oil instead of butter in cooking even if the portions didn't appear smaller for that particular week.

At first it might take one half hour or more before you and your partner are finished reviewing the journals, but this time will shorten.

As you begin to understand each other's habits, it will be easy to pin point patterns. Ideally, you'll be able to accomplish this in 15 to 20 minutes tops. The process needs to be time efficient for it to work long-term. Check the times that your partner ate. Did they go too long without eating between meals or snacks? Are they eating right before bed?

Also where did they eat? Was it riding in an elevator? Driving the freeway? Remember positive first. An example of the dialogue might go something like this; "I noticed you ate most of your meals sitting at your kitchen table, that's great. I also noticed that you ate a sandwich while riding on a rollercoaster. What happened here?" Granted this is an exaggeration, but it's an example of the way you might be able to approach the conversation. Your partner knew before you said anything that eating a sandwich on a rollercoaster was not a good idea, but the point is that you noticed it. You were engaged with what they were doing and you were really reading the journal. When we know that someone is going to be observing our habits, then it's easier to make more positive ones.

Look for patterns. Did you notice a nightly ice cream binge? Or perhaps daily visits to the vending machine at work? Remember, don't be punitive and say, "Why were you so weak that you couldn't stay away from the candy at work!" Instead try, "I noticed you used the vending machines quite a bit at work this week. Would it help to bring your own snacks to work? Let's say that your buddy doesn't like your solutions or suggestions. *Don't* be offended. Try to help them figure it out themselves.

Maybe they are going to the vending machine because they love chocolate. It's okay to love certain foods. Try and help them find an acceptable, lower calorie food that fits the bill so to speak. For instance, a 100-calorie snack of chocolate cookies or a single dark chocolate square instead of a jumbo sized candy bar from the vending machine.

Now it's your turn to have your journal read. There's no need to be defensive. Your buddy is there to help. Really listen to what they have to say. Chances are, you already know where you need to improve. Be gracious with comments. Also, accept the positive comments. Take those to heart. Build on the positive comments and really own them. This exchange during the journal reviews should be non-confrontational.

Advice should be given in a concerned way, and never punitive or scolding. You are there to help to each other and the longer you keep this up, the more it will help you. The following journal check-list will help you to remember certain things to look for when reviewing a journal. Don't expect your partner to include everything on list. It's a guide for you to use to provide kudos and to assist with making changes. Of course, the goal would be to have a diet that includes everything on the list, but this may take months to achieve. Take it in stride and make baby steps.

SUGGESTED FOOD JOURNAL CHECK LIST

(Based on The Dietary Guidelines for Americans 2010, recommendations from The American Heart Association, and The American Cancer Society)

Foods And Activities To Include:

- **5-7 total servings of fruits and non-starchy vegetables per day or 28 servings per week.** 1 serving of vegetable is equal to ½ cup cooked or 1 cup raw. 1 serving of fruit is about ½ cup cut-up or 1 whole piece (size of a baseball). Do not count the starchy vegetables like corn, peas, and potatoes in this category. Fruits and vegetables are high in vitamins, minerals, antioxidants, phytochemicals (may prevent cancer, heart disease, diabetes, and hypertension), and fiber. They are also lower in calories, fat, and sodium.
- **Fiber: 20-35 grams per day.** Fiber grams for whole grains can be found on the nutrition label. Fiber grams for fresh produce can usually be found on websites like Calorieking.com. Foods include 100% whole wheat bread, brown rice, alternate grains like wheat berry, spelt, and farrow. High fiber cereals (>6 grams fiber per serving), whole wheat pasta, beans, fruits and vegetables. The benefits include a decreased risk of diverticulitis, heart disease, and diabetes. They also promote regularity.
- **Healthy Fats (monounsaturated and polyunsaturated).** The **monounsaturated** fats can help to reduce bad cholesterol (LDL). They often are high in vitamin E.
- These fats are found in oils like olive, peanut, sesame, and sunflower. Good food sources include avocado, peanut butter, and most nuts and seeds. The **polyunsaturated** fats are found in many oils like corn, and safflower; they also reduce cholesterol and provide **omega-3** and **omega-6 fats.** These are essential fats that the body does not produce itself. Omega-3 fats are found in foods like salmon, tuna, sardines, shellfish, walnuts, flaxseed, and canola oil. Omega-6 is commonly found in most vegetable oils.
- **Nonfat or lowfat milk products.** This may include milk (non-fat or 1%), yogurt, kefir, cottage cheese, cheese, pudding, and ice cream. If available use organic products because these are produced without antibiotics, hormones, or synthetic chemicals.
- **Fluid intake:** 8 cups of water per day. There is no real consensus on how much water is required per day, but just count water and decaffeinated

beverages as your fluid. Fluid needs may vary with strenuous exercise, weather, and certain medications.
- **Fish:** 2 servings per week. For concerns about seafood contaminants and environmental issues go to **Seafoodwatch.org.** This site provides up to date information on the safest fish for consumption.
- **Exercise:** 120 minutes or more per week.
  Walk 10,000 steps per day. Measure steps with a pedometer. This is in addition to the 30 minutes of regular exercise. Get these extra steps by taking the farthest spots in parking lots, or climbing stairs for example.
- *FOODS TO LIMIT*
- **Avoid high sodium foods**; limit to 1500 mg day. Read labels. This may include foods with soy sauce or teriyaki sauce. Also canned foods, unless marked low sodium or no salt added. Watch for spice blends that contain salt, and packaged foods like boxed macaroni and cheese. Restaurant foods: look for the restaurant's nutritional information on-line for sodium content. Most flavored or sea salts still contain equivalent amounts of sodium to regular table salt.
- **Total Fat grams per day – not to exceed 30% of total calories.** You can also limit to 40 grams per day for women and 50 grams per day for men. The nutrition food label or Calorieking.com will provide this information.
- **High calorie beverages:** What other beverages are being consumed, including alcohol. How many calories are there, and what is the portion size? What for juices, sodas, and flavored milk.
  Fried foods: none, unless it's your birthday.
- **Avoid cured meats:** These are high in salt and nitrates. These are found mostly in foods like hot dogs, bacon, sausage, and lunchmeats.
- **Zero trans fats.** Food labels will list these. They are typically found in foods with hydrogenated oils. Keep in mind that a food may have up to ½ gram trans fat per serving even if the label is marked "0". Most tub or soft margarines no longer contain trans fats. Stick margarines do however, have them.

ADDITIONAL QUESTIONS TO ASK YOUR BUDDY

Portion size. What was the portion of food in relation to plate, glass or bowl size?

Food preparation style. How was the food cooked? Was it breaded, deep fried, or steamed? Preferably steamed, grilled, broiled, or baked. What type of fat, if any was used in cooking?

Were any extra condiments used? Condiments might include salad dressings, mayonnaise, cream cheese, sour cream, ketchup, barbeque sauce, butter, salt, etc.

Where was the food eaten? Was it in front of the television or driving in a car? Was your buddy distracted or eating too fast?

Lastly, you and your buddy should come up with your own items to review that pertain to your unique environments and circumstances.

SAMPLE FOOD JOURNAL

Hunger Scale: 1=Very Hungry 2=Hungry 3=Just Right 4=Full 5=Stuffed

Food & Portion Size	Time	Hunger	Exercise
1 CUP BRAN FLAKES, 1/2 CUP SKIM MILK, 1 BANANA, 1 CUP COFFEE WITH 2 TABLESPOONS UNSWEETENED CREAMER	6:30 A.M.	2	20 MINUTES WALKING ON TREADMILL

CHAPTER FIVE

PROGRESS

How do you know if your diet and weight loss efforts are successful? This can be done in a variety of ways. One way is to methodically measure your progress by some technique like weighing yourself. Or you can simply look in the mirror and see how you look and feel, or how your clothes fit. There's no right or wrong way to measure progress The no-measure method might be good for someone who may weigh themselves frequently, but becomes discouraged and gives up with minor unforeseen changes. Using the scale, weight circumference, or body fat analysis can be helpful for someone who is in denial about their habits. Either way, you should do some soul searching about what motivates you. You might want to try one method for a few weeks and jump to another if you're not sure.

THE SCALE

The scale can be your friend or your worst enemy. It doesn't always tell the truth, and most don't tell you how much body fat you may carrying. Try this; weigh yourself then get off the scale. Now drink a full glass of water and weigh yourself again. What happened? Try doing this while wearing different articles of clothing, shoes, jewelry etc. Do you see what I mean? The number on the scale can change as the wind blows. You want to look for overall trends in the scale and not just one weight measurement. If you weigh yourself through the day you will see different numbers as well. Think LOGICALLY about this. You did not gain fat by drinking the water, or by wearing different clothes. If you weighed at 7:00 a.m. and then again at 3:00 p.m. and weighed more, you didn't turn into a pumpkin - literally.

Fat change; gain or loss is much s-l-o-w-e-r than that. Use the scale as a tool, which is what it is for. Here are a few tips. Use the same scale when you weigh yourself. It could be your own scale, your buddy's scale, or even a scale at your gym. By using the same scale you are more likely to receive consistent results. People often weigh in at their doctor or dietitian's office and proclaim, "I swear, I lost weight on my scale at home, your scale is broken". Changes in the scale can also give you some insight into the sodium content of your diet. When someone has been monitoring their calories closely, and exercising but they gain *weight,* I always ask, "What did you eat yesterday, how many restaurants were you in, or did you have a lot of sushi with soy sauce. I ask those types of questions. Its almost 100% predictable that if you have a little more sodium in your diet than usual, you will see that number on the scale go up. This will make you crazy. This is where you can point out to your buddy that it's not fat gain, just water retention. Keep the positive reinforcement going. I know you want to blame yourself every step of the way for road blocks, but use this as an opportunity to learn a little bit more about how your body responds to different foods. Some people find it helpful to weigh themselves daily to keep themselves on track. I suggest in the beginning weigh once or twice a week. Friday is a great day to weigh because typically people are more consistent with their diet plans during the week. Weigh yourself at the same time of day and under the same conditions. For example; no clothes or jewelry, before eating or drinking anything, and after you've gone to the restroom.

This way you have a fair comparison. Also, use the same scale. Don't weigh yourself at home, then at the gym later, or at a friend's house after that. Again, ignoring consistent conditions would be another tactic to make you insane.

BODY FAT

To monitor body fat you can either do this yourself or go to a facility with more expensive equipment. Generally, women should be between 18-32% body fat. Men between 10-25% body fat. One technique is to measure skinfold thickness. For this, a device called a caliper is used. Essentially the skin and underlying fat are pinched at different sites on the body and measured. A caliper can be purchased on-line or in fitness stores and are relatively inexpensive. Another home method is the use of bioelectrical impedance. A hand held device or scale can be used. An electrical current is passed through the body to measure lean tissue. Height and weight are added and the percent body is calculated. Again, these devices can be purchased on-line or in fitness stores. The more costly and accurate methods for estimating body fat percentage are usually found at health spas, universities, research centers, and mobile units. These include hydrostatic underwater weighing, The Bod Pod (uses air), and DEXA (a type of xray). Just as I mentioned earlier with scales, try to use the same method of body fat percentage testing consecutively.

Another tool to measure change is with a tape measure. You can measure around your waist, your hips, thighs, arms etc. Another trick would be to use an unmarked piece a string without the numbers. Measure your beginning size and watch that string length increase as you shrink. Make sure you measure the same places each time and use body markers each time.

For instance if you are putting the tape measure around your thigh, find a freckle on your leg that you can pass the tape measure over each time to be consistent. Keep your focus on how good you feel. You're eating better, and getting more physical activity.

You should have more energy, more ambition, and more clarity of thought. Diet and exercise can provide immediate mental results. Focusing on those immediate "feel good" benefits can be more motivating than concentrating soley on the long-term benefits of weight loss. Blood chemistry or labs are another good way to measure progress. Total cholesterol and bad cholesterol (LDL) may decrease. Good cholesterol (HDL) may increase. You might also see a decline in blood glucose levels. Whether you have hypertension or not, your blood pressure will probably improve. All of these changes can occur from an improved diet, exercise, and weight loss. You may hear people say that you shouldn't lose more than 2 pounds per week because it would be unsafe to lose more than that at a time. That is somewhat true. You might only loose ½ pound per week, and I think that is great success. In the beginning you might lose 5 pounds the first week. That typically is not unsafe because it's partially water loss. Some weeks you might not lose anything. My point is that in this day and age with so many constraints that prevent us from losing weight, two pounds of weight loss per week for an extended period of time is nothing short of miraculous especially for women. Women have less body muscle than men and have to contend with life-long hormonal changes. Because weight loss is rarely a sustained linear decline, I suggest utilizing all the methods to monitor progress. For instance; weigh once or twice per week, measure waist circumference and/or other body parts once every other week, body fat percentage once per month, and check blood chemistry per your physician's recommendations.

CHAPTER SIX

MOTIVATION TO KEEP YOU GOING

In the beginning of any new weight loss program everything is great. You're pumped-up, and you feel like it will really happen this time. You do everything perfectly and follow the plan to the letter, then something happens. You run out of steam. You don't feel like paying attention to everything that you put into your mouth anymore. Exercise has become boring again. The scale is not moving as fast, or not at all. Now you want to quit and chalk it up to your inability to lose weight. You start to look at those ads in the back of magazines or late night infomercials for another weight loss miracle. You feel hopeless and out of control. This is a crucial moment in the process when you need to stop yourself and know that this lack of motivation is all normal. Most everyone hits this wall, which is why the weight loss industry is so huge. Every diet program out there knows you will get bored or quit, then eventually come back and try again. We tend to think first that we are the failure, not the program itself. This is the time to stop the pity party and pull out all of the stops. Before you start this weight loss endeavor it's a good idea to list all of the things that help motivate you. That way when you hit this wall, just look back on the motivator list you've created and pick one or all to keep you going. Your buddy and your food journal should remain your primary motivator. However, it's also good to add some new inspirations into the mix. So, now it's time to shake things up a bit. Here are a few suggestions for motivators and also ideas to distract you from eating, but please come up with as many as you can on your own.

1. Buy a trendy new piece of clothing that fits well (This may help you to feel good *now* and want to continue with the process).
2. Pull out of your closet a favorite piece of clothing that doesn't fit anymore, hang it somewhere visible so that you see it daily and often.
3. Take an unflattering *or* flattering picture of yourself and put it on the refrigerator or pantry door.
4. Listen to music all the time. Especially your favorite up beat dance music. Listen to it when your tired, exercising, or just need a lift.
5. Watch weight loss programs like The Biggest loser or Celebrity Fit Club. Or any of the health/fitness programs on The Learning Channel or Discovery Channels. Sometimes it helps to see other people who have the same struggles as you.
6. Find a favorite quote or slogan and put it on your bathroom mirror.
7. Spend more time with people who are health and fitness minded. If you don't know any, try to meet someone new, maybe at a gym class. (This is not a replacement person for your buddy).
8. Give yourself a boost with a new hair-style or color.
9. Call your buddy for support.
10. Hire a Registered Dietitian for a few sessions to help you keep on track.
11. Hire a personal trainer. Ask if you can get a reduced rate if you and your buddy go together.
12. Go to a day spa for a massage.
13. Take a walk in nature.
14. Take a fitness or dance class.
15. Volunteer or help someone out with a project, or be a good listener.
16. Browse the aisles of a health food store.
17. Take a healthy cooking class.
18. Learn a musical instrument or a new craft (keep your hands and mind busy).
19. Spend time at the library.
20. Start a weight loss support group.
21. Check out free health related lectures at your local hospital.
22. Visit a farmer's market.
23. Try a new recipe from a friend, a health oriented magazine or on-line.
24. Volunteer at your local hospital or free clinic (remind yourself of the benefits of good health).
25. Volunteer at the local animal shelter and walk a dog.

NEVER SAY NEVER

I think one of the biggest mistakes people make when trying to lose weight or even to change a lifestyle habit is to say, "I am *NEVER* going to eat that again" Also, people might say, "I am going to exercise every single day no matter what". That is a set-up for disappointment and a chance to "beat yourself up" again for failing.

It's unrealistic to think that you will never eat ice cream again when ice cream is actually your favorite food. (That would be me). Also, life happens and gets into the way of our exercise schedules. I had a client who was hosting her own child's birthday party. She served a delicious cake and ice cream. While everyone was enjoying the dessert, she decided to busy herself with clean-up and not indulge in the sweets.

She was very proud of herself for not eating the cake and ice cream, even though she was silently suffering. I did praise her for having the willpower not to indulge but thought she should have eaten some dessert anyway. This was a special occasion; it was her daughter's birthday. That would have been the time to indulge and not to feel guilty. It doesn't mean going hog-wild. She could have had just cake and no ice cream or she could have had cake and a little ice cream and not eat the frosting. That would have saved some calories for herself while showing her child how to eat "normally." I think it's important for your kids to see you have a healthy relationship with food and not always dieting or restricting. It would have been different if she didn't like cake and ice cream or had intolerances to them, but that was not the case.

It's one thing to completely give up something like alcohol, caffeine, or cigarettes because our bodies don't require those things. We need food for survival, there's no way around that. Of course we don't have to have cake and ice cream for survival, but they are also a part of socialization. They are fun. They are a treat. They can make us feel good when we're down or even better when we're up. Fun foods are not meant to be consumed daily, or instead of more nutritious foods. There's often a fine line to draw when food is involved. In this country we have become so all inclusive about food. "All or nothing" has become the mantra. We need to achieve balance to have healthy bodies as well as a healthy attitude about food.

The other part of this all or nothing mentality is exercise. We often over-analyze why we can't get motivated. We think there is a mental block, or again that maybe we need a shrink to help us figure it out. Look at it this way; when you start out as a couch potato, how can you realistically expect yourself to become an athlete overnight. It's like going from 0 to 60 mph in 5 seconds in a

Mini van. Just like the cliché of a baby learning to walk, it really is one step at a time.

MIND GAMES

There are many tricks we play with ourselves that prevent us from moving forward. Everyone thinks they are alone with the psychological mind tricks we play on ourselves. I am going to share with you just a few of those, and give you a few tips to counteract them.

Vacations and visitors are always dreaded by the person who is trying to lose weight. We assume that right in the midst of our hard work and motivation that everything will be ruined so that we'll have to start from square one.

For the person who is making serious life changes, the event (vacation or guests) goes by without much concern because there is typically more exercise due to sight-seeing. The problem is when the guests go home or we come home. Our taste buds are used to a different type of cuisine. We tell ourselves that we'll get back on track the day after or even the week after. Now you're back into the more sedentary lifestyle and it's easy to gain weight. It's important to enjoy the foods of different regions or treat your guests to your favorites but it's easy to continue with that mode of eating. Before the event occurs decide on a date that you will get back on track. Resume your program as soon as 24 to 48 hours. Actually decide what you'll be eating and schedule the physical activity to coincide. I think if you maintain your weight during a vacation or even gain a couple of pounds , you'll be in great shape!

We often think of dieting as an exercise of all or nothing – NO. We might think, "I will do this diet perfectly, or I will completely blow it". Think of this process as being on a train and headed for a particular destination. First you think about where you will go. You look at pictures or just imagine it. Next you purchase the ticket (you've made the commitment). Now you board the train. You're not sure where to sit, the people aren't familiar faces, you are a little unsure of what to expect but you are still excited with anticipation. Now you settle in. The scenery is beautiful. You have deep meaningful conversations with the other passengers. The food is delicious. You can't wait to get to the destination. After awhile you are disappointed to find the scenery doesn't change, the people are tedious, and the food is boring. You stop caring about the destination. The train now makes its first stop and you can't wait to get off. Now you're off the train for a few hours enjoying the change. The trains' whistle starts to blow.

The whistle reminds you that it's time to get back on. You can stay off the train and that is your choice. But, your ticket is still valid. The whistle is a reminder to get back on. It's not judging you that you took an hour break and got off. Some people got off and some people stayed. It is what it is. Now you can stay off the train and berate yourself by saying things in your head like, 'I will never get to my destination, there's something wrong with me for getting off the train, blah, blah blah". It doesn't make sense does it? You just get back on the train.

The whistle is just a friendly reminder that it's time. You might be surprised that by getting back on, that the scenery has changed, the food has been re-stocked and some of the people have changed. You might have a renewed outlook on what had become tedious. So now it's time to settle in and realize that depending where the destination is, it will be a slow ride. Sometimes you'll get off the train, other times you'll choose not to. Big deal – just get back on because the train will continue to get closer to the destination.

CHAPTER SEVEN

ADDITIONAL NUTRITION TIPS

FREQUENT EATING

Many people are often afraid to eat when they are trying to lose weight. They might not be hungry in the morning so they skip breakfast thinking, "Great, I'm saving calories!" Wrong. This is the worst approach. You aren't hungry in the morning partially because you're not used to eating at this time. Eating breakfast may not be a habit for you; and the anticipatory hormones and acids aren't flowing in your stomach getting ready for food. Remember that you haven't eaten for 12 plus hours, and now you expect to efficiently drive, work, raise kids, go to school, exercise, etc. Intellectually you know this a bad idea, and you're not really saving calories either. Here's why; your body is not going to burn calories as efficiently the next time you eat or use the fat on your body as quickly as it could. In fact things might slow down a bit. Your body starts to assume that you're living in a place with little to eat and famine conditions because there isn't a regular supply of food coming in, so your metabolism slows down a bit to reserve what you have stored. Your body has no idea that in reality everything is "Supersized". Eventually you will become hungry. In fact, you'll want to eat everything in sight. If you had only eaten earlier, you might have prevented this surge in appetite. Now you eat like a pig and after you're full, you say," Why did I do that? I know better than that. I have no self- control or I must be addicted to carbs, you say to yourself. Or you might consider that there was something from your childhood that's causing you to over-eat like this."

Wrong again. That behavior that feels like a vicious circle is totally normal. You didn't eat earlier, so now your body took over because you didn't have enough sense to feed yourself properly. When you are hungry you tend to eat faster, and it takes approximately 15 minutes for your brain to receive the signal that there is food in your stomach. That 15 minutes is a very long time of calorie consumption when you are eating fast. Now pair that truckload of calories with a slower metabolism (from not eating) and now you have a problem…weight gain!

Here's the trick; consume smaller portions, eat more frequently and dine slowly. This way you become satiated sooner and keep the calories at bay. Also this frequent eating might rev up your metabolism a little bit so that you can burn more calories at rest. Eat more often and lose weight. That seems like a pretty good deal to me!

Now you might say, "What about the extra calories from the in-between snacks"? Well, the snacks might help you increase your metabolism a little (thus burning more calories), and your body gets used to the fact there is a regular schedule of fuel coming in. It doesn't need to hang on to body fat so tightly. Most importantly, if the snack is balanced it should decrease the overload of calories eaten at the next meal. Anytime you feel "starving", there is a good chance that you'll eat too much and feel bad about it later. On a scale of 1 to 5, 1 being not hungry at all and 5 is very hungry, try to get to a point where you are only eating when you are between 3 and 4 on the scale.

Let's say conservatively that you consume 50 *less* calories during the day by having low calorie (100 or 200 calories) between meal snacks. This translates into 16,800 calories over the course of a year and then into 5 pounds of body fat.

Basically you are losing weight by eating more often, but hopefully not more calories overall. Also remember this isn't the only thing (exercise) you are doing to create a deficit in calories.

Typically you don't want to go longer than about 5 hours without eating. It takes a couple of hours for your food to fully digest and get into your blood stream, and then another few hours for your body to completely use this food for energy. If you can shorten this time between eating, that is ideal. Try to eat about every 3 or 4 hours at about the same times and see what happens. I guarantee you won't always be hungry when it's time to eat. Give it a try though, and after about a week or so you should start to feel hungry around those times you set aside to have meals or snacks. Don't force-feed yourself if you don't feel like eating; just have a little something like a few apple slices so that your body knows there's a constant supply of food coming in. Your body likes consistency when it comes to eating. Don't worry about the precise time that you eat. Go by your own schedule. You might hear people say not to eat past 7:00 p.m., but is that relevant if your dinnertime is 8:00 p.m. and you go to bed regularly at 12:00 or 1:00 a.m.? Don't split hairs about the exact time. Again, frequent and regularly timed meals and snacks should help with those evening binges.

STRUCTURE

Some people find they do better in the long run when they are not on a structured "program" for an extended period of time, and I tend to agree with this approach as a rule. Remember the name of the game is not to feel like you are on a rigid diet. Even though weight loss can be hard work, it shouldn't be tortuous. Going on a diet sets you up for going off of a diet and then back to old ways.

If you are starving yourself with a very restrictive diet and eating foods that you don't really enjoy then you might be constantly thinking about the day when you can eat the foods you ate before the diet. Instead of focusing on the future and how great you'll feel physically and mentally after the weight loss, the focus is on the past and deprivation. You then might start to think about how you are going to celebrate the weight loss. It could be with a food that is even more caloric than what you ate before the diet like a banana split, a double Cadillac margarita, or 5 servings of cheese macaroni and cheese. After the "celebration", you do it again on another day because you're still within range of your goal weight. Then you do it again and again. Now your taste buds, appetite, and habits have reverted back to the old ways and you've gained much of the weight back. Ideally, you should be learning how to fit the banana split into your life while you're losing weight. A modified version of a banana split that is. For example, It could be a smaller portion, have low fat ice cream, and fresh fruit instead of the sugary toppings. Your senses and psyche won't necessarily know the difference, and most importantly you won't be counting the days when it's all over. For our purposes here, we are going to throw in a little structure. Some structure can help you make those changes one step at a time. Structure and consistency will help to make those healthy behaviors become automatic. Basically, this is how to create new habits.

The first thing to do is set-up the times you are going to eat. Make sure these times are realistic with your lifestyle. Never go longer than 5 hours without eating. Try to be consistent. Now you might be whining that you're just not hungry in the morning or in the afternoon and can't eat. But I promise you, your appetite will adapt. Your body likes this consistency with eating. It's better to have small to moderate amounts of food continually rather than consuming large quantities once at the end of day. You should avoid feeling like your starving, especially in the evening. If you feel famished, then you are more likely to over eat at the next meal. Also you are more likely to pick at everything in the kitchen until dinner is ready, right? Those extra little bites that you take out of the pot or the refrigerator can add up to potentially hundreds of extra calories even before the meal begins. If you happen to be in a restaurant after a long day of restricting food, then the bread basket or chips will probably disappear. If you are never in a ravenous state, then you can avoid some of those extra calories.

Next determine your calorie needs. Most people will ask me (even strangers at a party), "How many calories should I be eating". Well, again there are several methods to figure this out. It's also very easy to over-estimate as well. Calorie needs are very individual. You have to consider your own metabolism. Are you someone who can sit down in a chair for an hour and not move one muscle. Or are you that person that sits down and can't stop moving. In each scenario, a different level of calories are burned. Also, consider your overall activity level. Do you use the stairs all day or are you a coach potato? Do you enjoy walking or running? Body composition of muscle and fat are also factored in. There are so many variables to include. As you can see, it's difficult to say how many calories someone needs off the top of my head.

SCREEN TIME

Stop wasting potential exercise time with television. We always have the excuse that our "favorite" show is on. After the hour show is over, we suddenly find a responsibility that calls us or we might get sucked into watching another show. Why not record your program and watch it during exercise or while you're making dinner, folding laundry, etc. It's also easy to lose time with the computer. You sit down to do some work or return emails and before you know it hours have been lost in cyberspace. I like to set a timer for a specified amount when I'm working on the computer.

It makes me more focused and more efficient. Practice good time management with screen time!

STOP CHEWING SO MUCH FAT

You hear so many conflicting theories about whether you should be eating fat or not. Then there is the mystery of good fat versus bad fat. Remember different approaches work for different people. I subscribe to the idea that less fat is better.

Yes, certain fats are considered "healthy". Examples include the Omega fatty acids which are found in foods like fish and flaxseed. Another example would be the monounsaturated fats that are high in olive or canola oil. Other fats are known as bad like transfats and saturated fats.

The problem that occurs is that people have a false sense of security about the "good" fats. A cardiologist may say, "eat almonds, they are good for your heart". Yes that's true because they have monounsaturated and omega fats. The reality of how that message translates into the real world is that people will buy large bags of almonds and eat them by the handfuls. Other people, and you know who you are, will buy bags of dark chocolate almonds telling themselves that the antioxidants from the dark chocolate is even better. The problem with this rationale is that nuts have calories.

If you are gaining weight because of too many calories, then you have negated the benefit from the nuts. Ten medium sized almonds are approximately 100 calories. A handful for me is about 20 nuts. And let's face-it, if there's a bag of nuts open at home its easy to eat several handfuls while telling ourselves, "it's healthy".

I believe a good way to eat nuts, walnuts or almonds is to eat a few chopped-up on hot cereal or in salads. If you can truly limit yourself to 10-12 at a time as a designated snack then go for it. I have a friend, Paul who portions himself 10 almonds in a baggy and brings them to work for a snack. He is very lean and this works for him. If I tried that, I'd eat several on the side as I was portioning the nuts in the bag. A trick I use, is that I tend to buy walnuts. I don't like walnuts that much so I'm not as tempted to over eat them.

The Buddy System Diet

Quick Tips on Sodium

It's easy to forget about the sodium content in foods when you're trying to focus on so many other things like calories, fat, fiber, and exercise. But sodium is one thing that can quickly put a wrench in your motivation. Too much sodium can make you retain fluid, causing the scale to soar. You can see the pounds increase by up to five pounds in one day despite careful attention to exercise and calories. Bloating from extra water weight will even make you *feel* FAT. Besides the psychological damage added salt can do, it can increase your risk for heart disease and stroke.

The biggest problem with sodium is that its hidden everywhere. People who don't use the salt shaker often feel that they don't get any added sodium to their diet. Of course avoiding extra added salt is important, but the majority of sodium comes from processed and restaurant foods. The American heart association recommends limiting your daily sodium intake to less than 1,500 milligrams per day. Just one teaspoon of table salt contains 2,000 milligrams!

What is the difference between salt and sodium? Salt is a generic term used for many other chemicals and sodium happens to be one of them. We use the term salt when referring to a compound in food. That is sodium chloride. Sodium may be paired with other chemicals like sodium bicarbonate, monosodium glutamate, etc. Sodium is the mineral we are concerned with and it really only tastes "salty" when combined with chloride. Don't use your taste buds as a guide to whether a food is high in sodium. Read food labels, go to websites, and restaurant guides to look up the sodium content.

For example the sodium from a popular fast-food restaurant shows the regular cheeseburger as containing 680 milligrams of sodium and the small french fries as having 160 milligrams of sodium. We instinctively think the fries would have more sodium because we taste the sprinkled salt directly on our tongues. The burger has sodium incorporated in the meat, the cheese, and the bread.

Lastly don't be fooled into thinking that sea salt or any other gourmet salts have less sodium. The difference is primarily in the grain and the taste. Take a look at the label and you will see. Having said that, sometimes we use less of a larger grain salt, which is a good thing.

Overall, do your best to eliminate as much sodium as possible by limiting canned soups, breads, cheese, cured meats, and condiments like soy sauce. Instead use fresh herbs, garlic powder, lemon juice, or flavored vinegars.

Additional Nutrition Tips

WHAT TO EAT

We talked about how important planning and preparation are to your success. Because you are extraordinarily busy, I have prepared some menus for you. I've also included recipes as well. If you don't like something, just switch it out for something of similar nutritional value and/or calories. For example, if the menu has an apple you can exchange that for an orange. Don't make it too complicated. Don't stress if the calories aren't exactly the same. There are so many variables in nature any way, that the calories listed for fresh fruits and vegetables are typically averages.

    I think one of the biggest challenges for people is trying to figure what to eat for dinner. You may have worked all day and at 4:00 you finally start thinking about to have. By this time in the day your options are either too labor intensive to think about preparing. You don't have any groceries at home. Possibly you hate to cook and the other options are mostly unhealthy restaurant foods. This is why I wanted to take some of thinking out of it for you. I would bring you the groceries if I could.

    I know it's a reality that you won't always have time to plan the weeks' meals out all the time. That is where the recipe cards come in handy. The cards are meant to be kept in your glove box, purse, or desk drawer. If its 4:00 with nothing planned, you can grab the cards and take them to the grocery store. The ingredients are right there for simple dinners.

CHAPTER EIGHT

MOVE IT LIKE JAGGER

This current top hit is a great way to think about exercise. Let's face it; most people do not enjoy exercise. We can find hours and hours of time to do other tasks like emptying a closet that has been full for ten years or watching hours of television. It's amazing how there's never an hour of extra time to exercise. But, if we make exercise more of a natural way of moving (like Jagger), we can burn more calories without having to carve out a chunk of time during our already hectic days. Some people call this the "fidget factor". You know, you see people who tap their feet, squirm in their chair, move their hands when talking, or pace when talking on the phone. All of these activities burn more calories than not. Over time the calories add up to hundreds or even thousands of calories consumed over the course of a year. That's what I mean by "Move it like Jagger."

Most people's thoughts about exercise need an attitude shift. Believe me, I can relate. I think there are several ways to look at it. First, of course there are the health benefits. Regular physical activity can lower blood pressure, normalize blood sugars, reduce risk for cancer and heart disease, etc. Lastly, it can help with intestinal health, bone density, depression, and weight loss. When someone points out those long-term health benefits, as I just did, we often think initially it's interesting and important. But, we also might subconsciously disregard the importance because there isn't an immediate pay off. When there isn't an immediate reward, then we aren't usually as motivated. Especially where weight loss is concerned. So instead of struggling to figure out how to embrace something that we don't want to think about in the future, shift the thinking to the immediate pay-off of exercise.

Because there are many quick benefits. Forget about exclusively embracing the long term benefits to our health. Of course, those are the most important reasons for exercising. but the reality is that humans go back for more when there is an immediate pay off to how we feel or even instant results that are measurable. I believe the coffee market would be sparse if it wasn't for the instant "pick-me-up" factor!

One enticing immediate benefit of physical activity is that your mood will improve right after a work-out. I can't tell you how many times I've been down, or frustrated and after thirty minutes on the treadmill, my mood was transformed. The effects will last for hours.

Regular activity can also improve your concentration. Many work environments are actually purchasing treadmill desks so the employees can walk and do work at the same time. Studies have shown that we work more efficiently under these circumstances. My own physician even uses an under-the-desk pedal exerciser which he uses while dictating.

Some people find that regular activity improves sleep. And sleep, as we now know is related to obesity. When we become sleep deprived hormones change in our bodies that help regulate hunger and satiety. Thus leaving us feeling hungrier and not knowing when to stop eating. Also, when we lack sleep, we are left too tired to exercise which starts a vicious cycle of not exercising.

Self esteem is elevated after physical activity. Whether it's a walk around the park or the completion of a marathon, it always feels good to be responsible and to take care of ourselves. The competitive nature of a race can also drive us to keep training, and to keep improving. There's nothing like that feeling of accomplishment!

For a diabetic, exercise can reduce blood glucose levels and the effects can last up to 24 hours. Of course, talk to your doctor first before starting any type of exercise program.

Hopefully I've sold you on the idea of doing regular exercise. Now here is another the problem; how to be consistent. This is where your buddy can help.

On our own, we can often muster up the willpower to do some regular activity for a few days. After that, the excuses start to pile up for not doing it. Consequently we start to feel bad about ourselves then all activity comes to a screeching halt. We begin to avoid the thought of exercising. If we bought a new gym membership, we start to feel like too much time has passed since we were there, then we avoid the place all together. (Gym's make their profits from people who don't go). The mind games we play with ourselves are endless.

I believe there are two key ingredients for consistent exercise. The first one is to make the activity social. You have your buddy already there. When exercise becomes a social event, it's easier to show up and it's much more fun while you do it. The activities you can share with your buddy are endless.

On the next page I've listed many types of activities to try. I suggest doing something you've never tried before. Maybe take a class or even share the cost of a personal trainer. If your buddy lives in another city, you can still check in with him/her and report your exercise in your journal. Give each other the same encouragement as you would with the diet.

The other important component is to make yourself an appointment to exercise. We all know how to keep appointments, even if it's for ourselves. If you wake up in the morning and tell yourself that you're going to exercise sometime during the day it won't happen. Too many distractions get in the way. If you designate a certain time to exercise on a calendar with the rest of your appointments, then its easier to work your other activities around that. Don't forget to factor in the extra time that revolves around the activity itself. For instance; drive time, change of clothing, special equipment, etc. You and your buddy could incorporate exercise the same day you review the journals as well.

It's more important to do 20 minutes of exercise daily rather than become overwhelmed with a time commitment you can't realistically keep and then do nothing at all. Over time the habit will develop and it will be easier to add more time and frequency to your workout. An easy way to make that appointment is by finding a class of some sort like Zumba or spinning. The class meets at regular times and it's social. So remember; make it social and make an appointment. Lastly, check with your doctor to see if there are any restrictions to certain types of exercise.

IDEAS FOR NEW FITNESS ACTIVITIES

Walking
Hiking
Jogging
Rock Climbing
Swimming
Rowing
SCUBA Diving
Snorkeling
Water Skiing
Water Aerobics
Surfing
Ballroom Dancing
Line Dancing
Clogging
Ballet
Zumba
Fencing
Horseback Riding
Jump Rope
Hula Hoop
Mountain Biking
Karate
Judo
Tai Chi
Yoga
Pilates
Skiing/Snow Boarding
Racquetball
Tennis
Squash
Golf
Bowling
Ice Skating
Roller Skating

1200 CALORIE PLAN

This plan is basically the same as the 1500 calorie plan, but with a few smaller portions and asmaller snack between lunch and dinner. Also, there isn't a night time snack You shouldn't be hungry on this plan. If you find yourself anxious to eat anything around you; wait about 15-20 minutes. This is called "riding the wave of hunger". The hunger will pass. Try to drink some water or a low calorie beverage and distract yourself with some kind of activity for those 15 minutes. Take your dog for a walk, fold laundry, or pay bills! you can also add more vegetables to your meals and snacks.

SAMPLE SCHEDULE:

Breakfast:
7:00 AM
200 calories

Snack:
9:30-10:30 AM
100 calories

Lunch:
12:00-1:00 PM
400 calories

Snack:
3:00-4:00 PM
100 calories

Dinner:
6:00-7:00 PM
400 calories

1200 CALORIE PLAN
BREAKFAST SUGGESTIONS
200 CALORIES

Egg sandwich: 1 egg white (microwave approximately 35 seconds) 1 toasted whole wheat English muffin (100 calories) 1 slice low-fat cheese (about 50 calories) 1 slice tomato or 1 tablespoon salsa & ½ orange (or apple) & black coffee or black tea or water with lemon	**NOTES:** Can assemble as a sandwich or scramble the egg with cooking spray and top with cheese and salsa.
Cold cereal: High fiber cereal (7 grams per serving or more) – about ½ cup or 100 calories & ½ cup skim or nonfat milk & ½ banana & coffee or tea or water	**NOTES:** Can use ½ cup berries (any kind) instead of the banana.
Hot cereal: ½ cup unsweetened cooked oatmeal & ½ cup chopped apple & 1 tablespoon chopped walnuts & 1 tsp brown sugar & ¼ cup skim/nonfat milk & coffee or tea or water	**NOTES:** Can substitute the apple for 1 tablespoon raisins or cranberries

1200 CALORIE PLAN
LUNCH SUGGESTIONS
400 Calories

Cold Sandwich: 2 slices 100% whole wheat bread (about 100 calories per slice) 3 ounces turkey (prefer reduced sodium and nitrate free) Vegetables – any amount and be creative (cucumber, shredded carrots, spinach, tomato, onion, etc.) Mustard and/or 1 tsp light mayonnaise & 1 apple or 1 cup of grapes & sparkling or still water	**NOTES:** Can exchange the turkey for 3 oz. tuna or skinless chicken breast. Many sandwich chains offer nutrition information in the store or online. Look for sandwiches with a total of 300-350 calories.
Frozen Entrée: 1 entrée. Look for brands with 400 mg sodium or less. Organic options are often available. 300-350 calories for the entire meal. & 1 apple (or 1 pear, 1 orange, 1 peach, or 1/2 banana) & sparkling or still water	**NOTES:** Healthier brands are often found next to the frozen soy or vegetarian items. It's good to have food in the freezer for back-up. Fresh food is always better, but these foods are portione controlled and typically less calories than restaurant foods.
Hot Sandwich: 2 slices 100% whole wheat bread (100 calories each slice or less) 1 slice low-fat cheese (approximately 50 calories) Grill without butter in an indoor grill or in a skillet with cooking spray. & 1 cup low sodium tomato soup & sparkling or still water	**NOTES:** Add sliced tomato, onion or any vegetable to sandwich for flavor and volume. Can substitute tomato for low sodium vegetable soup.

1200 CALORIE PLAN
DINNER SUGGESTIONS
400 Calories

Extra Lean Protein: 5 ounces grilled white turkey, tofu, white fish, or 8 medium size shrimp. ½ baked sweet potato with butter spray 1 cup steamed spinach (flavor with 1-2 tsp apple cider vinegar) 100 calories of a healthy fat (either for cooking or condiment) – example 2 tsp olive oil, or 2 tsp margarine, etc. sparkling or still water	**NOTES:** This is a filling meal if you're very hungry. Can substitute ½ regular potato with skin for the sweet potato.
Pasta or Rice Main Dish: 1 cup whole wheat pasta (cooked) with ½ cup turkey bolognaise sauce (recipe) **OR:** 3/4 cup cooked brown rice with 3 ounces extra lean protein (see above) 1 cup mixed vegetables steamed (broccoli, carrots & cauliflower) with 1 tsp parmesan cheese or margarine sparkling or still water	**NOTES:** If using regular white pasta, use ¾ cup cooked. Save time by steaming fresh precut, or frozen vegetables in the microwave.
Meat Craving: 3 ounces cooked boneless beef filet or boneless pork loin 1 cup Savory Cauliflower (recipe) 1 cup green salad with 2 tablespoons low-fat dressing of choice. Sparkling or still water	**NOTES:** Best choice is grass fed organic beef. Can substitute cauliflower for any other steamed green vegetable like asparagus, broccoli, or green beans. Use any type of salad greens and any non-starchy vegetables.

1500 CALORIE PLAN

This plan is basically the same as the 1200 calorie plan, but with a few larger portions and a more substantial snack between lunch and dinner. You shouldn't be hungry on this plan. If you find yourself anxious to eat anything around you; wait about 15-20 minutes. This is called "riding the wave of hunger". The hunger will pass. Try to drink some water or a low calorie beverage and distract yourself with some kind of activity for those 15 minutes. Take your dog for a walk, fold laundry, or pay bills!

SAMPLE SCHEDULE:

Breakfast:
7:00 AM
300 calories

Snack:
9:30-10:30 AM
100 calories

Lunch:
12:00-1:00 PM
400 calories

Snack:
3:00-4:00 PM
200 calories

Dinner:
6:00-7:00 PM
400 calories

Snack:
7:00-8:00 PM
100 calories

1500 CALORIE PLAN
BREAKFAST SUGGESTIONS
300 CALORIES

Egg sandwich: 2 egg whites (microwave approximately 35 seconds) 1 toasted whole wheat English muffin (100 calories) 1 slice low-fat cheese (about 50 calories) 1 slice tomato or 1 tablespoon salsa & 1 whole orange (or apple) & black coffee or black tea or water with lemon	**NOTES:** Can assemble as a sandwich or scramble the egg with cooking spray and top with cheese and salsa.
Cold cereal: High fiber cereal (7 grams per serving or more) – about 1 cup or 200 calories & ½ cup skim or nonfat milk & ½ banana & coffee or tea or water	**NOTES:** Can use ½ cup berries (any kind) instead of the banana.
Hot cereal: 1 cup unsweetened cooked oatmeal & ½ cup chopped apple & 1 tablespoon chopped walnuts & 1 tsp brown sugar & ¼ cup skim/nonfat milk & coffee or tea or water	**NOTES:** Can substitute the apple for 1 tablespoon raisins or cranberries

1500 CALORIE PLAN
LUNCH SUGGESTIONS
400 Calories

Cold Sandwich: 2 slices 100% whole wheat bread (about 100 calories per slice) 3 ounces turkey (prefer reduced sodium and nitrate free) Vegetables – any amount and be creative (cucumber, shredded carrots, spinach, tomato, onion, etc.) Mustard and/or 1 tsp light mayonnaise & 1 apple or 1 cup of grapes & sparkling or still water	**NOTES:** Can exchange the turkey for 3 oz. tuna or skinless chicken breast. Many sandwich chains offer nutri-tion information in the store or online. Look for sandwiches with a total of 300-350 calories.
Frozen Entrée: 1 entrée. Look for brands with 400 mg sodium or less. Organic options are often available. 300-350 calories for the entire meal. & 1 apple (or 1 pear, 1 orange, 1 peach, or 1 nectarine) & sparkling or still water	**NOTES:** Healthier brands are often found next to the frozen soy or vegetarian items. It's good to have food in the free-zer for back-up. Fresh food is always better, but these foods are portioned controlled and typically less calories than restaurant foods.
Hot Sandwich: 2 slices 100% whole wheat bread (100 calories each slice or less) 1 slice low-fat cheese (approximately 50 calories) Grill without butter in an indoor grill or in a skillet with cooking spray. & 1 cup low sodium tomato soup & sparkling or still water	**NOTES:** Add sliced tomato, onion or any vegetable to sandwich for flavor and volume. Can substitute tomato for low sodium vegetable soup.

1500 CALORIE PLAN
DINNER SUGGESTIONS
400 Calories

Extra Lean Protein: 5 ounces grilled white turkey, tofu, white fish, or 8 medium size shrimp. ½ baked sweet potato with butter spray 1 cup steamed spinach (flavor with 1-2 tsp apple cider vinegar) 100 calories of a healthy fat (used for cooking or condiment) – example 2 tsp olive oil, or 2 tsp margarine, etc. sparkling or still water	**NOTES:** This is a filling meal if you're very hungry. Can substitute ½ regular potato with skin for the sweet potato.
Pasta or Rice Main Dish: 1 cup whole wheat pasta (cooked) with ½ cup turkey bolognaise sauce (recipe) **OR:** 3/4 cup cooked brown rice with 3 ounces extra lean protein (see above) 1 cup mixed vegetables steamed (broccoli, carrots & cauliflower) 1tsp parmesan cheese or margarine sparkling or still water	**NOTES:** If using regular white pasta, use ¾ cup cooked. Save time by steaming fresh pre-cut, or frozen vegetables in the microwave.
Meat Craving: 3 ounces cooked boneless beef filet or boneless pork loin 1 cup Savory Cauliflower (recipe) 1 cup green salad with 2 tablespoons low-fat dressing of choice. sparkling or still water	**NOTES:** Best choice is grass fed organic beef. Can substitute cauliflower for any other steamed green vegetable like asparagus, broccoli, or green beans. Use any type of salad greens and any non-starchy vegetables for salad.

1700 CALORIE PLAN

This plan shouldn't leave you hungry but still can provide results. You have some flexibility here with the meals and snacks. You can add some calories to the beginning of the day by decreasing from later in the day. It's always better to consume more calories earlier in the day and decrease as the day goes by if possible. It's still important not to skip a meal or snack entirely even if you are rearranging your calories.

SAMPLE EATING SCHEDULE:

Breakfast:
7:00 AM
300 calories

Snack:
9:30-10:30 AM
200 calories

Lunch:
12:00-1:00 PM
500 calories

Snack:
3:00-4:00 PM
200 calories

Dinner:
6:00-7:00 PM
400 calories

Snack:
7:00-8:00 PM
100 calories

1700 CALORIE PLAN
BREAKFAST SUGGESTIONS
300 CALORIES

Egg sandwich: 2 egg whites (microwave approximately 35 seconds), 1 toasted whole wheat English muffin, 1 slice low-fat cheese, 1 slice tomato or 1 tablespoon salsa 1 whole orange (or apple) black coffee or black tea or water with lemon	**NOTES:** Can assemble as a sandwich or scramble the egg with cooking spray and top with cheese and salsa. Have the English muffin or 2 corn tortillas on the side.
Cold cereal: High fiber cereal (7 grams per serving or more) – about 1 cup or 200 calories ½ cup skim or nonfat milk ½ banana coffee or tea or water	**NOTES:** Can use ½ cup berries (any kind) instead of the banana.
Hot cereal: 1 cup unsweetened cooked oatmeal ½ cup chopped apple 1 tablespoon chopped walnuts 1 tsp brown sugar ¼ cup skim/nonfat milk coffee or tea or water	**NOTES:** Can substitute the apple for 1 tablespoon raisins or cranberries

1700 CALORIE PLAN
LUNCH SUGGESTIONS
500 Calories

Cold Sandwich: 2 slices 100% whole wheat bread (about 100 calories per slice), 3 ounces turkey (prefer reduced sodium and nitrate free), vegetables – any amount and be creative (cucumber, shredded carrots, spinach, tomato, onion, etc.), mustard and/or 1 tsp light mayonnaise 1 apple or 1 cup of grapes 12 almonds sparkling or still water	**NOTES:** Can exchange the turkey for 3 oz. tuna or chicken breast. Many sandwich chains offer nutrition information in the store or online. Look for sandwiches with a total of 300-350 calories.
Frozen Entrée: 1 entrée, 400 mg sodium or less, 300-350 calories for the entire meal. 1 apple (or 1 pear, or 1 orange, or ½ banana) 1 cup Greek salad (recipe) sparkling or still water	**NOTES:** Healthier brands are often found next to the frozen soy or vegetarian items.
Hot Sandwich: 2 slices 100% whole wheat bread, 1 slice low-fat cheese. Grill without butter in an indoor grill or in a skillet with cooking spray. 1 cup low sodium tomato soup 1 banana sparkling or still water	**NOTES:** Add sliced tomato or onion to sandwich for flavor and volume. Can substitute for low sodium vegetable soup.

1700 CALORIE PLAN
DINNER SUGGESTIONS
400 Calories

Extra Lean Protein: 5 ounces grilled white turkey, tofu, white fish, or 8 medium size shrimp. ½ baked sweet potato with butter spray 1 cup steamed spinach (flavor with 1-2 tsp apple cider vinegar) 100 calories of a healthy fat (used for cooking or condiment), example 2 tsp olive oil, or 2 tsp margarine, etc. sparkling or still water	**NOTES:** This is a filling meal if you're very hungry. Can substitute ½ regular potato with skin for the sweet potato.
Pasta or Rice Main Dish: 1 cup whole wheat pasta (cooked) with ½ cup turkey bolognaise sauce (recipe) **OR:** 3/4 cup cooked brown rice with 3 ounces extra lean protein (see above) 1 cup mixed vegetables steamed (broccoli, carrots & cauliflower) with 1 tsp parmesan cheese or margarine sparkling or still water	**NOTES:** If using regular white pasta, use ¾ cup cooked. Save time by steaming fresh pre-cut, or frozen vegetables in the microwave.
Meat Craving: 3 ounces cooked boneless beef filet or boneless pork loin 1 cup Savory Cauliflower (recipe) 1 cup green salad with 2 tablespoons low-fat dressing of choice. sparkling or still water	**NOTES:** Best choice is grass fed organic beef. Can substitute cauliflower for any other steamed green vegetable like asparagus, broccoli, or green beans. Use any type of salad greens and any non-starchy vegetables for salad.

RECIPES

APPETIZERS

- Artichoke Dip
- Salt Free Pickles
- Eggplant Dip
- Stuffed Jalapenos
- VegetableCceviche
- Tzadiki

SOUPS

- Gazpacho
- Corn Chowder
- Curried Carrot
- Lentil
- Red Hot Chili
- Carrot and Corn
- Tomato Florentine
- Vegetarian Cabbage Stew
- Vegan Mushroom

SALADS

- Chopped Greek
- Crunchy Chicken
- Garden
- Southwestern
- Veggie-Tuna

SIDES

- Delicious Green Beans
- Savory Cauliflower
- Stuffed Peppers

MAIN

- A Whole Lotta Eggs
- Cesear Salad With Scallops
- Corn And Crab Enchiladas
- Oven Fried Fish
- Greek Chicken
- Turkey Burgers
- Garden Pizza
- Grilled Salmon
- Jalapeno-Pineapple Chicken
- Chicken Piccata
- Lemony Halibut
- Pesto Pasta
- Light Lasagna
- Pork And Mango
- Spicey Snapper
- Summertime Pasta
- Tandoori Chicken
- Turkey Bolognaise
- Turkey Stroganoff
- Zesty Rice and Chicken

DESSERT

- Berry Cheesecake
- Cherry Crisp
- Flourless Chocolate Orange Cake
- Strawberry-Mango Gazpacho
- Tropical Punch Parfait

ARTICHOKE DIP

This can be served as a side dish by leaving the artichoke hearts whole.

INGREDIENTS:

1 tablespoon olive oil

2 garlic cloves minced

1 pound frozen artichoke hearts thawed and chopped finely

2 tablespoons fire roasted diced green chilies (canned)

1/2 cup fat-free low sodium chicken broth

1/4 teaspoon red pepper flakes

1/3 cup panko bread crumbs

1/3 cup parmesan cheese grated

Olive oil cooking spray

DIRECTIONS:

Heat the olive oil in a deep skillet and saute the garlic for approximately 1 minute. Add the artichoke hearts, chilies, pepper flakes, salt to taste. Cook until the artichokes begin to brown. Pour ingredients into a baking dish. Sprinkle the top evenly with panko crumbs and parmesan cheese. Liberally spray the top with cooking spray. Bake in a 450 degree oven for about 10 minutes.

NUTRITION:

6 Servings

Calories: 95

Fat: 4 grams

Sodium: 161 milligrams

Carbohydrate: 10 grams

Fiber: 5 grams

Protein: 4 grams

SPEEDY SALT FREE PICKLES

This makes a great low calorie appetizer or snack

INGREDIENTS:

5 pickling cucumbers cut into 1/2 inch rounds or 3 regular peeled and sliced

2 cups white vinegar

2 cups water

3 tablespoons pickling spice

2 tablespoons sugar

2 garlic cloves sliced

2-3 sprigs fresh dill

DIRECTIONS:

Combine vinegar, water, spices, garlic, sugar , and bring to a boil. Pour over cucumbers in a glass bowl and add dill. Refrigerate at least 1 hour.

NUTRITION:

Approximately 6 servings

Calories: 38

Sodium: 3 milligrams

Fat: 0

Carbohydrate: 9 grams

Fiber: 1 gram

Protein: 1 gram

TUNA STUFFED JALAPENOS

This recipe sounds odd, but it tastes delicious. My friend Lori always made this for me and I always refused to try it. When I finally did, it was a hit.

INGREDIENTS:

6 ounces albacore tuna rinsed

1/2 medium carrot finely diced

1/4 cup red onion finely diced

1 tablespoon light mayonnaise

3 tablespoons sweet pickle relish

1 tablespoon cilantro finely diced

Approximately 12 pickled jalapenos sliced lengthwise and seeded

INSTRUCTIONS:

Mix together the tuna, carrots, cilantro, relish, onion, and mayonnaise. Stuff the jalapeno halves with approximately 2 teaspoons of the tuna mixture. Refrigerate for about 1 hour. Garnish with a cilantro sprig.

NUTRITION:

Per each jalapeno half

Calories: 29

Fat: 1 gram

Sodium: 49 milligrams

Carbohydrate: 2 grams

Fiber: 0

Protein: 4 grams

GREEK STYLE TZADIKI DIP

This sauce can also be used on burgers or served with fish.

INGREDIENTS:

4 garlic cloves minced

4 tablespoons red onion minced

8 ounces light sour cream

1/2 cucumber skinned, seeded, and diced

1 tablespoon fresh dill finely chopped

1 tablespoon fresh mint finely chopped

1 teaspoon lemon zest

White pepper and salt to taste

DIRECTIONS:

Mix all ingredients well and refrigerate at least one hour. Serve with vegetable sticks or baked pita chips.

NUTRITION:

4 Servings

Calories: 89

Fat: 6 grams

Sodium: 42 milligrams

Carbohydrate: 7 grams

Fiber: 0

Protein: 2 grams

VEGETABLE CEVICHE

INGREDIENTS:

1/2 cucumber peeled and seeded, diced finely

1 large tomato seeded and diced

1 cup jicama peeled and diced

1/2 cup red onion diced

1/2 cup cilantro chopped finely

2 tablespoons lime juice

4 tablespoons lemon juice

2 cloves garlic minced

1/2 jalapeno seeded and diced finely

1 teaspoon chili powder

1/2 teaspoon cumin

Fresh ground pepper

Salt to taste

DIRECTIONS:

Combine all ingredients and refrigerate overnight. Serve with baked tortilla chips or as a salad.

NUTRITION:

4 servings

Calories: 30

Protein: 1 gram

Fat: 0

Carbohydrate: 7 grams

Fiber: 3 grams

Sodium: 6 milligrams

CORN CHOWDER

This is just a good cozy soup

INGREDIENTS:

1/2 white onion chopped

1 teaspoon olive oil

14 ounces fat-free and low sodium chicken broth

2 russet potatoes peeled and diced

2 celery stalks chopped

1 cup water

1 1/2 cups fresh yellow corn

1/2 cup parsley stems removed finely chopped

1 cup non-fat milk

Ground pepper and salt to taste

DIRECTIONS:

Sauté onion in oil until soft. Add the chicken broth until simmering. Add the potatoes and celery. When the potatoes are soft puree the mixture but leave the potatoes a little chunky. Mix in the water, corn, and parsley. On low heat slowly add the milk and serve.

NUTRITION:

Approximately 6 servings

Calories: 118

Fat: 2 grams

Sodium: 176 milligrams

Carbohydrate: 25 grams

Fiber: 2 grams

Protein: 4 grams

SOUTHWEST CARROT AND CORN SOUP

INGREDIENTS:

1 medium yellow onion chopped

1/2 green bell pepper chopped

14 ounces low sodium vegetable broth

3 cups water

5 medium carrots peeled and diced

1 jalapeno seeded and diced

3 cups no salt added diced tomatoes drained

2 cups yellow corn (fresh or frozen)

2 tablespoons cilantro finely chopped

1/4 teaspoon mace

4 corn tortillas cut into 1/4 inch strips

1 lime

2 teaspoons paprika

Cooking spray

DIRECTIONS:

Saute the onion and bell pepper in 1/4 cup broth until the onion is clear. Add the remaining broth, 2 cups water, carrots, and jalapeno. Boil until the carrots are soft. Add the tomatoes, corn, cilantro, mace, pepper, salt to taste, and remaining water. Simmer on low for about 10 to 15 minutes. Spray a baking sheet with cooking spray then place the tortilla strips without overlapping. Sprinkle the strips with lime juice and paprika. Bake at 350 degrees for about 10 minutes or until crunchy.

NUTRITION:

    Calories: 85

    Fat: 1 gram

    Sodium: 80 grams

    Carbohydrate: 19 grams

    Fiber: 4 grams

    Protein: 2 grams

ANYTIME LENTIL SOUP

Serve this soup as an appetizer or main dish at lunch or dinner

INGREDIENTS:

2 cups dried lentils

4 cups water

1 yellow onion chopped

1 tablespoon olive oil

3 garlic cloves minced

1/2 green bell pepper seeded and diced

1 celery stalk diced

1/4 cup dry white wine

3 Roma tomatoes diced

2 teaspoons dried parsley flakes

DIRECTIONS:

Saute onion in olive oil until soft. Add garlic and celery and cook about 1 minute. Add remaining ingredients and cook for about 40 minutes.

NUTRITION:

Approximately 8 servings

Calories: 204

Fat: 2 grams

Sodium: 9 milligrams

Carbohydrate: 32 grams

Fiber: 15 grams

Protein: 13 grams

KARL'S RED HOT CHILI

This recipe is in memory of my dear friend Karl Klessig

INGREDIENTS:

1/2 red onion diced

1/2 teaspoon olive oil

2 garlic cloves minced

1 red bell pepper diced

1 pound lean turkey Italian sausage, casing removed and cubed

28 ounces no salt added stewed tomatoes

8 ounces no salt added tomato sauce

2 tablespoons chili powder

1/2 teaspoon oregano

1/2 teaspoon cumin

16 ounces low sodium kidney beans

Hot pepper sauce

Fresh ground pepper

DIRECTIONS:

Saute the onion, bell pepper, and garlic in olive oil until soft. Add turkey and cook until browned. Add stewed tomatoes, tomato sauce, chili powder, oregano, and cumin and cook for about 15 minutes. Add the beans and cook for another 5 to 10 minutes. Add pepper sauce and pepper to taste.

NUTRITION:

Approximately 5 servings

Calories: 325

Protein: 25 grams

Fat: 12 grams

Carbohydrate: 35 grams

Fiber: 11 grams

Sodium: 584 milligrams

TOMATO-CARROT FLORENTINE SOUP

The best of both worlds. Green and red, lots of nutrition!

INGREDIENTS:

6 ounces no salt added tomato paste

1 small russet potato peeled and cubed

1 small onion diced

2 garlic cloves minced

14 ounces fat-free low sodium chicken broth

2 cups water

1 1/2 cups fresh spinach chopped

1 tablespoon fresh basil finely chopped

4 tablespoons balsamic vinegar

1/2 teaspoon garlic powder

Fresh ground pepper to taste

DIRECTIONS:

In a large stockpot combine the tomato paste, potato, onion, garlic, chicken broth, and water. Cook until the potato becomes very soft. Turn the stove off and puree the ingredients with an immersion blender. Add the remaining ingredients and cook until the spinach becomes limp.

NUTRITION:

Approximately 6 Servings Carbohydrate: 13 grams

Calories: 65

Fat: 0

Sodium: 155 milligrams

Protein: 2 grams

VEGETARIAN SWEET AND SOUR CABBAGE STEW

I love sweet and sour soup, but I'm not crazy about the chunks of beef. You can add the beef to this recipe

INGREDIENTS:

8 cups Water

1 head Green cabbage chopped (about 4 cups)

3 stalks Celery chopped

2 cups Carrots peeled and chopped

1 Yellow onion chopped

1 cup White wine vinegar

1 and 1/2 teaspoons dried tarragon

2 tablespoons fresh parsley chopped

1/4 teaspoon white pepper

2 Russet potatoes with skin diced

3 tablespoons white sugar

DIRECTIONS:

Combine all of the ingredients in a large pot and simmer partially covered for about 2 hours or until the potatoes are soft. The vinegar and sugar can be adjusted to your taste.

NUTRITION:

Approximately 8 servings

Calories: 86

Protein: 2 grams

Fiber: 3 grams

Sodium: 45 milligrams

VERY VEGAN MUSHROOM SOUP

A hearty soup, but it can be eaten any time of the year

INGREDIENTS:

2 shallots minced

1 teaspoon olive oil

2 garlic cloves minced

5 large Italian mushrooms chopped

1/2 cup sherry

2 1/4 cups water

1/2 russet potato skin on cubed

1 cup fresh parsley chopped

3 green onions chopped

Fresh ground pepper to taste

Salt to taste

DIRECTIONS:

Sauté the shallots in olive oil until soft. Add the garlic and cook for about 30 seconds. Add 1/4 cup water, mushrooms, sherry, pepper, and salt. Cook for about 7 minutes. Add the remaining water, onion, parsley, and potato. Cook until the potato is soft and puree. Garnish with minced parsley.

NUTRITION:

Serves 4

Calories: 70

Fat: 1 gram

Sodium: 15 milligrams

Carbohydrate: 9 grams

Fiber: 2 grams

Protein: 2 grams

CHOPPED GREEK SALAD

This is a refreshing salad that can be served as an appetizer or main dish.

INGREDIENTS:

4 cups romaine lettuce chopped

1 cup arugula chopped

3/4 red onion finely chopped

1/2 cup parsley finely chopped

4 ounces reduced fat feta cheese

2 tablespoons fresh oregano coarsley chopped

1 cup roasted red peppers finely chopped

8 ounces artichoke hearts packed in water chopped

1/4 cup pitted kalamata olives chopped

15 ounces low sodium garbanzo beans rinsed

2 tablespoons fresh basil chopped

1 tablespoon olive oil

Juice from 1/2 lemon

1 teaspoon lemon zest

2 tablespoons red wine vinegar

1/2 teaspoon garlic powder

Salt and Pepper to taste

DIRECTIONS:

Combine the oil, lemon juice, lemon zest, vinegar, garlic powder, pepper, and salt. Mix well. Combine the remaini ng ingredients with the dressing. Toss well and serve.

NUTRITION:

Approximately 8 servings

Calories: 110

Fat: 4 grams

Sodium: 557 milligrams

Carbohydrate: 15 grams

Fiber: 4 grams

Protein: 6 grams

Recipes

CRUNCHY CHICKEN SALAD

This recipe can be used for salads or sandwiches

INGREDIENTS:

2 Boneless chicken breasts with skin

Juice from 1 lemon divided in half

Fresh ground pepper

1/2 Red onion diced

1/2 Green apple diced

1/2 cup Red grapes cut in half

1 stalk celery diced

1/8 cup Walnuts chopped

1 tablespoon Dijon mustard

2 tablespoons light mayonnaise

4 cups mixed green lettuce chopped coarsely

DIRECTIONS:

Pre-heat oven to 400 degrees. Place chicken on baking sheet drizzle with 1/2 lemon juice and ground pepper to taste. Bake for about 15 minutes minutes on each side or when fully cooked. After co oking, place chicken in refrigerator for about 1 hour or more. Remove skin and cut into 1/2 inch cubes and place in a large bowl. Add the remaining ingredients to the bowl except lemon juice. Mix ingredients together and serve on lettuce. Drizzle with remaining juice and fresh pepper.

NUTRITION:

Serves 4

211 calories

10 grams carbohydrate

10 grams fat

100 milligrams sodium

3 grams fiber

16 grams protein

CRUNCHY GARDEN SALAD

Any kind of lettuce leaves can be used in this salad. I used romaine because of the crunchy texture.

INGREDIENTS:

2 cups Broccoli florets

6 cups Romaine lettuce, cut into bite size pieces

8 Cherry tomatoes halved

10 Baby carrots halved

1 cup Sugar snap peas

1 Red bell pepper cut into 1 inch strips

4 Stalks green onion cut into 1 inch strips

1 cup low sodium Kidney beans (canned) rinsed

1 cup Shredded low fat mozzarella cheese

2 tablespoons Olive oil

6 tablespoons Balsamic vinegar

Juice from 1 whole lemon

Fresh ground pepper to taste

DIRECTIONS:

Steam broccoli in microwave for about 90 seconds. Mix in a large bowl broccoli, lettuce, tomatoes, carrots, peas, bell pepper, onion, beans, and cheese. In a separate bowl mix together the oil, vinegar, and lemon juice. Drizzle the dressing into the salad and toss the ingredients well. Serve and top with fresh ground pepper.

NUTRITION:

6 Servings

Calories: 219

Protein: 18 grams

Fat: 10 grams

Carbohydrate: 15 grams

Fiber: 7 grams

Sodium: 343 milligrams

CALIFORNIA SOUTHWESTERN SALAD

INGREDIENTS:

1 cup fresh (or defrosted from frozen) corn

3/4 cup fresh cilantro chopped, stems removed

1 bunch green onions chopped

2 tomatoes chopped

1 green bell pepper chopped

2 cups romaine lettuce chopped

2 chicken breasts skinless boneless grilled and finely chopped

3/4 cup fat free ranch dressing

1 cup garbanzo beans rinsed

4 or more dashes hot pepper sauce

1 cup baked tortilla chips crushed

DIRECTIONS:

Mix all ingredients well and top with tortilla chips.

NUTRITION:

4 Servings

Calories: 282

Fat: 4 grams

Sodium: 610 milligrams

Carbohydrate: 43 grams

Fiber: 7 grams

Protein: 20 grams

PUMPED UP TUNA SALAD

You can add more veggies to this salad. Add whatever is leftover in your refrigerator

INGREDIENTS:

7 ounces low sodium albacore tuna packed in water

1/4 red onion chopped finely

1 medium tomato seeded and diced

1 stalk celery chopped finely

1 cup broccoli florets diced finely

1 tablespoon Dijon mustard

1 tablespoon lite mayonnaise

DIRECTIONS:

Mix all ingredients together. Chill for 1 hour and serve on a bed of spring greens

NUTRITION:

(Based on 2 servings)

Serves 2-4

Calories: 198

Protein: 31

Fat: 5 grams

Carbohydrate: 9 grams

Fiber: 3 grams

Sodium: 328 milligrams

MY FAVORITE GREEN BEANS

This dish is super simple but company worthy

INGREDIENTS:

12 ounces steam in the bag frozen whole green beans

1 tablespoon Dijon mustard (or to taste)

1 teaspoon dried tarragon

White pepper and salt to taste

INSTRUCTIONS:

Cook the green beans per bag instructions. While still hot mix the green beans with the remaining ingredients.

NUTRITION:

Serving size 1 cup

Calories: 43

Fat: 1 gram

Sodium: 91 milligrams

Carbohydrate: 5.94 grams

Fiber: 2.04 grams

Protein: 1.32 grams

SAVORY CAULIFLOWER

INGREDIENTS:

1 head cauliflower cut into 1 inch pieces

3 cloves garlic crushed

1 tablespoon olive oil

3 tablespoons white wine vinegar

1/2 cup dry white wine

1/2 tsp cumin

1/2 tsp paprika

DIRECTIONS:

Saute garlic in olive oil for about 1 minute and then add cauliflower. Cook for about 2 minutes. Add the remaining ingredients and cook until the liquid has evaporated.

NUTRITION:

4 servings

Calories: 90

Fat: 3.5

Protein: 3 grams

Carbohydrate: 8 grams

Sodium: 43 milligrams

Fiber: 3 grams

VEGETARIAN STUFFED BELL PEPPERS

INGREDIENTS:

2 green bell peppers seeded and halved lengthwise

2 cups fresh spinach chopped

1/2 cup no salt added diced tomatoes drained

1/4 cup mozzarella cheese shredded

1 tablespoon fresh tarragon

2 tablespoons toasted pine nuts

Ground pepper to taste

DIRECTIONS:

Pre-heat oven to 350 degrees. Mix together the spinach, tomatoes, cheese, tarragon, pine nuts, and pepper. Divide equally and fill the bell pepper halves. Place peppers in a baking dish filled with 1/2 inch water. Cover and bake until the peppers are soft.

NUTRITION:

Serves: 4

Calories: 89

Fat: 5 grams

Sodium: 138 milligrams

Carbohydrate: 6 grams

Fiber: 2 grams

Protein: 5 grams

Recipes

A WHOLE *LOTTA* EGGS

This is a very filling meal and great for a quick dinner. Any type of vegetables can be substituted.

INGREDIENTS:

1 dozen egg whites (crack and separate or use equivalent egg substitute)

2 cups frozen mixed bell peppers

14 ounces diced tomatoes no salt added, drained

1 teaspoon garlic powder

4-5 fresh basil leaves or 1/2 teaspoon dried

1 teaspoon olive oil

2 tablespoons grated parmesan cheese

Salt and pepper to taste

DIRECTIONS:

Whisk together the eggs and set aside. In a large skillet saute the bell peppers in olive oil for approximately 5 minutes or until most of the water has evaporated. Add the tomatoes and cook another 5 minutes. Add the garlic, basil, and eggs. Scrape the sides of the skillet with a spatula as the eggs are cooking as you would with scrambled eggs. When the eggs are firm remove from heat. Sprinkle with parmesan cheese, salt and pepper.

NUTRITION:

2 servings

Calories: 213

Protein: 25 grams

Fat: 4 grams

Carbohydrate: 11 grams

Fiber: 4 grams

Sodium: 455 milligrams

CAESAR SALAD WITH SCALLOPS

Salmon or chicken can be used instead of the scallops

INGREDIENTS:

3 sourdough rolls cut into 8ths

1 teaspoon olive oil

1 teaspoon paprika

1/4 teaspoon kosher salt

1/2 teaspoon garlic powder

1/2 cup low fat buttermilk

Juice from 2 lemons

1 teaspoon dry mustard

3 garlic cloves minced

1/2 teaspoon anchovy paste

1 teaspoon Worcestershire sauce

1 ounce fresh parmesan cheese grated

2-3 drops hot pepper sauce

1 pound jumbo scallops

1/4 cup orange juice

1 lime

2 heads Romaine lettuce torn into bite size pieces

DIRECTIONS:

Croutons
Place roll pieces, oil, 1/2 teaspoon paprika, garlic powder, and salt in a large zip lock bag. Shake bag vigorously until the bread is covered evenly. Place bread on a baking sheet that has been sprayed with cooking spray. Bake at 250 degrees until crisp.

Dressing

Whisk together the buttermilk, lemon juice, anchovy paste, mustard, garlic, pepper sauce, Worcestershire sauce, and parmesan cheese. Combine the dressing, and croutons with the lettuce.

Scallops

Mix the orange juice, lime juice, 1/2 teaspoon paprika and pour over scallops in a baking dish. Cook for about 15 minutes on the broil setting or until browned.

Assembly

Divide salad onto 4 plates. Divide scallops evenly and place on top of the salad.

NUTRITION:

Calories: 325

Fat: 7 grams

Sodium: 532 milligrams

Carbohydrate: 40 grams

Fiber: 8 grams

Protein: 30 grams

CORN AND CRAB ENCHILADAS WITH VERDE SAUCE

This dish was based on a favorite at the restaurant Casa Vega in Studio City, California

INGREDIENTS:

10 corn tortillas

1 pound tomatillos

2 garlic cloves minced

1 Serrano chili seeded and finely minced

3 tablespoons lime juice

1/3 cup canned Ortega chilies diced

2 green onions chopped

1/2 cup cilantro chopped

1 teaspoon white sugar

1/4 teaspoon salt

1/2 teaspoon olive oil

1/2 yellow onion finely diced

1 cup corn fresh or frozen

1/2 pound lump crabmeat

1/2 cup nonfat sour cream

Ground pepper to taste

DIRECTIONS:

Pre-heat oven to 400 degrees. Peel paper skin from the tomatillos. Boil the tomatillos whole for about 10 minutes. Drain the water then puree the tomatillos in a blender or food processor. Add garlic, lime juice, chillies, onions, salt, cilantro, and sugar. Puree mixture again and set aside. Heat oil in a large skillet, add the onions and cook until soft. Add the corn, crab meat, sour cream, and ground pepper. Cook the mixture until heated thoroughly. Wrap the tortillas in aluminun foil and place in the oven for about 15 minutes to soften. Spray a casserole dish with nonstick spray. Place 1/4 cup of the crab mixture in the center of each tortilla and roll up. Place in the casserole dish. Pour the tomatillo mixture over the enchiladas. Bake uncovered for about 20 minutes or until sides bubble.

NUTRITION:

2 enchiladas per serving

Calories: 247

Fat: 3 grams

Sodium: 298 milligrams

Carbohydrate: 40 grams

Fiber: 3 grams

Protein: 16 grams

CRISPY OVEN FRIED FISH

This goes well with any type of salsa or tomato based sauce.

INGREDIENTS:

4 Filets of white fish (e.g. snapper, tilapia, orange roughy)

1 cup Japanese Panko bread crumbs

2 tablespoons flour

3 egg whites lightly beaten

1/4 cup nonfat milk

1/2 teaspoon paprika

1/4 teaspoon Kosher salt

Fresh ground pepper to taste

DIRECTIONS:

Pre-heat oven to 450 degrees. Mix the Panko crumbs with the flour, paprika, salt, and pepper. In a separate bowl lightly beat the egg whites and milk. Dip each fish filet into the egg mixture, then into the bread crumbs and coat well. Place each fish filet on a baking sheet that has been sprayed with cooking oil. Spray and coat each filet as well. Cook for about 10 minutes or until the fish turns white.

NUTRITION:

Serves 4

Calories: 180

Protein: 28 grams

Fat: 2 grams

Carbohydrate: 14 grams

Sodium: 91 milligrams

SUPER SIMPLE GREEK STYLE CHICKEN

Serve this dish with a salad or green vegetable.

INGREDIENTS:

3/4 cups uncooked brown rice

1 10 ounce can low sodium low fat cream of chicken condensed soup

1 1/3 cups water

1 tsp dried oregano

Zest from whole lemon

Juice from 1/2 lemon

1 clove garlic minced

6 chicken thighs boneless and skinless

3 1/2 ounces low fat feta cheese crumbled

DIRECTIONS:

Pre-heat oven to 375 degrees. Combine all of the ingredients except the feta cheese in a baking or casserole dish. Cover and cook for about 60 minutes. Remove from oven and sprinkle with feta cheese.

NUTRITION:

6 Servings

Calories: 217

Fat: 6 grams

Sodium: 488 milligrams

Carbohydrate: 204 grams

Fiber: 1 gram

Protein: 19 grams

GARDEN PIZZA

You can use your favorite pizza crust. I like this one because it comes out thin and crispy.

INGREDIENTS:

1 package Pillsbury Pizza Crust

6 ounces no salt added tomato paste

2 cloves garlic crushed

1 tablespoon balsamic vinegar

2 tablespoons water

1 tablespoon parmesan cheese

1/2 teaspoon sugar

1/2 teaspoon dried oregano

1/2 teaspoon dried basil

2-3 drops hot pepper sauce

1 cup part skim mozzarella cheese grated

1 cup green bell pepper diced

1/2 cup white onion diced

2 Roma tomatoes chopped

1 zucchini un peeled diced

1 cup sliced mushrooms

DIRECTIONS:

Pre-heat oven to 350 degrees. Combine tomato paste, garlic, vinegar, water, parmesan cheese, sugar, oregano, basil, and pepper sauce and cook for about 10 minutes. Prepare pizza crust per manufacturer directions. Spread the tomato sauce evenly onto the uncooked dough. Evenly sprinkle the mozzarella cheese on top of the sauce. layer the remaining ingredients evenly. Cook the pizza for about 25 minutes or until the edges of the crust become golden brown.

NUTRITION:

1/6 of the pizza

Calories: 321

Fat: 9 grams

Sodium: 800 milligrams

Carbohydrate: 43 grams

Fiber: 4 grams

Protein: 21 grams

CANADIAN STYLE BAKED SALMON

INGREDIENTS:

12 ounces fresh salmon cut into 3 ounce portions

1 tablespoon olive oil

1 tablespoon Dijon mustard

1 tablespoon orange zest

2 tablespoons maple syrup

2 tablespoons lemon juice

Ground black pepper to taste

Salt to taste

DIRECTIONS:

Pre-heat oven to 450 degrees. Salt and pepper salmon to taste and place skin side down in a baking dish. Combine remaining ingredients then brush onto salmon evenly. Cook salmon for approximately 15 minutes.

NUTRITION:

4 Servings

Calories: 238

Fat: 14 grams

Sodium: 145 milligrams

Carbohydrate: 8 grams

Fiber: 0

Protein: 19 grams

JALAPENO-PINEAPPLE CHICKEN

INGREDIENTS:

4 4 ounce chicken breasts boneless and skinless

2 egg whites lightly beaten

1/2 cup fat free milk

1 1/2 cups corn flakes gently crushed

1 tablespoon all-purpose flour

1 tablespoon brown sugar

1 teaspoon nutmeg

1 cup fresh pineapple finely chopped

1 green bell pepper seeded and diced

2 medium tomatoes seeded and diced

1 jalapeno seeded and finely diced

1/2 cup cilantro chopped

1/2 red onion finely diced

1 tablespoon white vinegar

Salt and Pepper to taste

INSTRUCTIONS:

Pre-heat oven to 350 degrees. Combine the eggs and milk, set aside. In another bowl mix the corn flakes, flour, brown sugar, nutmeg, salt, and pepper. Dip the chicken in the egg wash, then the corn flake mixture. Cover both sides of the chicken well. Spray a baking sheet with cooking spray and lay the chicken flat. Spray each chicken breast as well and cook for about 30 minutes or until done. Combine the pineapple, bell pepper, tomatoes, jalapeno, cilantro, onion, and vinegar. Refrigerate until ready to serve with the chicken.

NUTRITION:

4 servings

Calories: 205

Fat: 2 grams

Sodium: 130 milligrams

Carbohydrate: 19 grams

Fiber: 2 grams

Protein: 28 grams

LEMONY CHICKEN PICCATA

This is one of my favorite quick and easy dishes.

INGREDIENTS:

8 ounces plain nonfat yogurt

4 skinless boneless chicken breast (approx 4 ounces each)

1/2 cup flour

1 teaspoon paprika

1 tablespoon olive oil

1 teaspoon margarine

2 cloves garlic minced

Juice from 1/2 lemon

1 cup white vermouth

1/2 cup lemon juice

1/2 cup water

2 tablespoons capers drained

Salt and pepper to taste

DIRECTIONS:

Marinate chicken overnight in yogurt. Rinse chicken and pat dry. Mix together flour, paprika, salt and pepper. Dip the chicken in flour mixture and cover both sides. On medium-high heat, brown the chicken on both sides in the oil, margarine, and juice from 1/2 the lemon. Reduce heat and cook until done. Set the chicken aside on a plate and keep warm. Scrape the brown bits from the pan and add garlic, 1/2 cup lemon juice, vermouth, 1/2 cup water, and capers. Cook the liquid and reduce by half. Add the chicken back into the pan and simmer for about 3 minutes.

NUTRITION:

4 servings

Calories: 316

Protein: 30 grams

Fat: 6 grams

Carbohydrates: 20 grams

Fiber: 1 gram

Sodium: 260 milligrams

LIGHT AND FLAKEY LEMONY HALIBUT

In a pinch any type of meaty white fish can be used instead of halibut.

INGREDIENTS:

1 filet halibut (approximately 10-11 ounces)

1 large lemon, 1/2 thinly sliced (about 6 slices), juice from other half

1 teaspoon dried oregano

1/8 th cup lowfat feta cheese crumbled

DIRECTIONS:

Pre-heat oven to 350 degrees. Spray baking dish with olive oil spray. Lay 3 lemon slices in the baking dish. place the fish on top of the lemon slices. Lightly spray the fish with oil spray. Sprinkle the fish with oregano. Lay the remaining lemon slices on top of the fish. Bake for about 20 minutes uncovered, or until the fish turns white and flakey. Sprinkle the fish with lemon juice and feta cheese before serving.

NUTRITION:

2 servings

Calories: 255

Protein: 45 grams

Fat: 7 grams

Carbohydrate: 0

Fiber: 0

Sodium: 306 milligrams

LIGHT AND FRESH PESTO PASTA

This recipe first appeared in an issue of Muscle and Fitness *Hers*

INGREDIENTS:

1 1/2 cup fresh basil chopped

6 cloves garlic crushed

1/2 cup walnuts chopped

1/2 cup parmesan cheese grated

1/4 cup olive oil

1/4 cup water

1 pound box high protein penne pasta

1/2 medium raw zucchini chopped

1/2 large tomato chopped

1 teaspoon balsamic vinegar

DIRECTIONS:

Combine the basil, garlic, walnuts, cheese, olive oil and water by adding one at a time to a blender or food processor. Cook the pasta as directed by manufacturer. Add 1 cup of the pesto mixture to the hot pasta and mix well. Mix together the tomatoes, zucchini, and vinegar. Top each serving of pasta with 1/4 cup of the tomato mixture.

NUTRITION:

4 servings

Calories: 643

Fat: 27 grams

Sodium: 236 milligrams

Carbohydrate: 71 grams

Fiber: 8 grams

Protein: 25 grams

LIGHT AND LUSCIOUS LASAGNA

This dish is a little more labor intensive, but it's great for leftovers.

INGREDIENTS:

1/2 brown onion finely diced

1 teaspoon olive oil

3 garlic cloves minced

5 ounces low fat breakfast sausage finely chopped

3 1/2 cups spaghetti sauce

2 tablespoons balsamic vinegar

2 cups fat free cottage cheese

2 egg whites

1/4 teaspoon nutmeg

Ground pepper

1 cup zucchini shredded

1 cup low fat mozzarella cheese shredded

12-14 fresh basil leaves

2 cups sliced mushrooms

1 cup fresh spinach leaves

1/2 eggplant thinly sliced crosswise

12 sheets of no-bake lasagna pasta

2 tablespoons parmesan cheese grated

DIRECTIONS:

Pre-heat oven to 350 degrees. In a saucepan heat oil and cook onions until soft, then add garlic. Add sausage and cook until browned. Add spaghetti and vinegar until heated. Set aside. Mix together the cottage cheese, egg whites, nutmeg, and pepper. Set aside. Mix together the zucchini and mozzarella cheese. Set aside. In the bottom of a 9 x 13 inch pan spread 1 cup of the tomato sauce evenly. Lay 3 sheets of pasta on the sauce without overlapping. Layer 1/2 cup of cottage cheese mixture evenly, then layer the basil leaves evenly. Next layer the mushrooms and follow with 1 cup of sauce. Layer 1 cup of cottage cheese mixture, then 3 sheets of pasta. Layer the remaining cottage cheese, then the eggplant. Layer 1 cup sauce, then the zucchini mixture. Layer the remaining cottage cheese. Layer the spinach evenly and top with remaining zucchini mixture. layer the remaining pasta and sauce. Sprinkle with parmesan cheese. Bake covered for 35 minutes. Uncover and cook for another 20 minutes or until bubbly.

NUTRITION:

8 servings

Calories: 311

Fat: 10 grams

Sodium: 507 milligrams

Carbohydrate: 34 grams

Fiber: 3 grams

Protein: 20 grams

PORK LOIN CHOPS WITH MANGO SALSA

If mango is not available, then pineapple can be substituted

INGREDIENTS:

4 1 inch thick boneless pork loin chops

1 medium whole mango peeled and diced

2 tablespoons fresh cilantro chopped

4 tablespoons lime juice

1 tespoon red chili powder

DIRECTIONS:

Sprinkle pork with salt and pepper as desired, and roast at 350 degrees for approximately 20 minutes. In a separate bowl mix the remaining ingredients. Divide the salsa evenly and serve with the pork.

NUTRITION:

Per Serving, 4 servings

208 calories

25 grams protein

55 milligrams sodium

7 grams fat

8 grams carbohydrate

1 gram fiber

EASY SPICY SNAPPER

This is a great dish for people who *don't* love fish.

INGREDIENTS:

2 filets of Red Snapper (or any light white fish) fresh or thawed

1 jar mild no sodium red salsa

1 bag frozen green beans

DIRECTIONS:

Pre-heat oven to 350 degrees. Mix greens and salsa in a casserole dish. Lay fish on top of the mixture and cover. Bake for 20 minutes or until the fish is white and flakey.

NUTRITION:

2 servings

Calories: 218

Protein: 25 grams

Fat: 1.5 grams

Carbohydrates: 31 grams

Fiber: 9 grams

Sodium: 130 milligrams

FORTIFIED TURKEY BURGERS

Don't tell anyone there's spinach in these burgers!

INGREDIENTS:

1 pound extra lean ground turkey

4 tablespoons uncooked old fashioned rolled oats

4 tablespoons finely diced walnuts

1 tablespoon worcestershire sauce

1 cup raw spinach chopped

DIRECTIONS:

Roast the oats and walnuts in a saucepan on the stovetop for about 2-3 minutes, set aside. Mix together the turkey, spinach, worcestershire sauce, walnuts, and oats. Make 4 patties about 4 inches across. Cook the patties in a counter-top grill for about 5 minutes.

NUTRITION:

(analysis without bread)

4 servings

Calories: 202

Fat: 6 grams

Protein: 28 grams

Carbohydrate: 8 grams

Sodium: 76 milligrams

TANDOORI STYLE CHICKEN

I Love Indian food! This is a super easy version of a traditional Indian dish

INGREDIENTS:

- 1 cup nonfat plain yogurt
- 1/2 cup fat free half and half
- 5 garlic cloves crushed
- 1 tablespoon lemon juice
- 1 teaspoon ground coriander
- 1 teaspoon tumeric
- 1 teaspoon ground cumin
- 1/2 teaspoon ground cloves
- 1 teaspoon chili powder
- 1 tablespoon paprika
- 2 pounds boneless skinless chicken breasts

DIRECTIONS:

Combine and mix all the ingredients except the chicken. Cut the chicken into 3 ounce portions, then cut 1/2 inch down the middle of each piece. Place the chicken in the yogurt mixture and refrigerate overnight. Take the chicken out of the yogurt mixture and bake for about 30 minutes in a 425 degree oven.

NUTRITION:

(per 3 ounce serving)
Calories: 202
Protein: 28 grams
Carbohydrate: 15 grams
Fat: 1 gram
Fiber: 0
Sodium: 209 milligrams

TURKEY BOLOGNAISE

This is a very basic classic recipe. It can even be eaten without the carbohydrates.

INGREDIENTS:

1 pound mild or sweet Italian turkey sausage, with casing removed

3 garlic cloves minced

28 ounces no salt added chopped tomatoes with juice

1/4 cup balsamic vinegar

1/2 cup red wine

1/4 cup parmesan cheese grated

DIRECTIONS:

Spray a deep skillet with cooking spray. Brown the turkey while breaking up to resemble ground meat. Add remaining ingredients and simmer on low heat for about 30 minutes. Serve with brown rice or whole wheat pasta.

NUTRITION:

(without rice or pasta)

About 5 servings

Calories: 258

Fat: 11 grams

Sodium: 654 milligrams

Carbohydrate: 10 grams

Fiber: 2 grams

Protein: 25 grams

TURKEY STROGANOFF

Another classic recipe, but a favorite

INGREDIENTS:

1 pound lean ground turkey

1 white onion chopped

4 cups sliced brown mushrooms

1 can low fat low sodium condensed cream of mushroom soup

1/2 cup dry red wine

1 teaspoon dried tarragon

Fresh ground pepper to taste

1/4 cup fresh parsley chopped

DIRECTIONS:

Spray a deep skillet with cooking spray and brown the turkey. Add the onion and cook until soft. Add mushrooms and cook for about 2 minutes. Add wine, soup, ground pepper and simmer for approximately 20-30 minutes. Remove from heat and fold in the sour cream. Serve over yolkless noodles or brown rice. Sprinkle with parsley.

NUTRITION:

approximately 5 servings

(Calculated without noodles or rice)

Calories: 225

Fat: 8 grams

Sodium: 235 milligrams

Carbohydrate: 15 grams

Fiber: 1 gram

Protein: 19 grams

ZESTY RICE AND CHICKEN

This recipe takes about an hour to make, but it's super tasty!

INGREDIENTS:

4 Boneless skinless chicken breasts

1 tablespoon olive oil

1/2 juiced lemon

Fresh ground pepper

3 Large carrots peeled and chopped

1 Yellow onion diced

1 red bell pepper diced

3 Cloves garlic crushed

1/4 teaspoon cayenne pepper

1 and 1/2 cups Brown rice

2 cups Low sodium chicken broth

1 tablespoon Lemon zest

1 teaspoon oregano

1/2 cup Dry white wine

Fresh Cilantro sprigs for garnish

DIRECTIONS:

In a large pan brown the chicken in olive oil, lemon juice, and pepper for about 4 minutes on each side. Take chicken out of the pan and set aside. Add onion to the pan and cook until soft. Add carrots, red pepper, cloves, and cayenne pepper; cook for about 2 minutes. Stir in the rice and cook for another 2 minutes. Add the chicken broth, lemon peel, oregano, and wine. Cover the pan and simmer for about 40 minutes or until the rice is fully cooked. Add the chicken and cook for about 5 minutes or until fully cooked. Garnish with cilantro and serve.

NUTRITION:

4 Servings

calories: 331

protein: 31 grams

fat: 8 grams

Sodium: 222 milligrams

Carbohydrate: 26 grams

Fiber: 4 grams

REDUCED FAT BERRY CHEESECAKE

This recipe is based on my mom's scrumptious cheesecake recipe.
She's the best cook in the world.

INGREDIENTS:

1 1/2 cups cinnamon flavored low fat graham crackers crushed (about 10 rectangles)

1 tablespoon brown sugar packed

1 1/2 tablespoons margarine melted

1 1/2 teaspoon Tahitian vanilla extract

24 ounces reduced fat Neufchatel cheese

1 cup fat free sour cream

1 cup liquid egg substitute

4 tablespoons fresh lemon juice

1 1/2 teaspoons grated lemon rind

1 cup low fat buttermilk

1 1/3 cups and 1 teaspoon ultrafine granulated sugar

1/2 cup sliced strawberries

1/2 cup blueberries

1/2 cup raspberries

1 tablespoon brandy extract

DIRECTIONS:

Mix graham crackers, brown sugar, margarine, and 1/2 teaspoon vanilla. Press evenly into the bottom of a 9" spring form pan. Chill for about 30 minutes. Gently beat the Neufchatel cheese, sour cream, egg substitute, lemon juice, and lemon rind until smooth. Fold in the buttermilk, 1 and 1/3 cups sugar, and 1 teaspoon vanilla. Pour ingredients into pan and place in a 350 degree pre heated oven for 1 hour, then chill. Mix the berries, brandy extract, and 1 teaspoon sugar. Spread berry mixture over cake before serving.

NUTRITION:

16 servings

Calories: 230

Sodium: 279 milligrams

Fat: 10 grams

Carbohydrate: 28 grams

Fiber: 1 gram

Protein: 7 grams

STRAWBERRY- MANGO GAZPACHO

This is a light dessert. Serve in a fancy glass

INGREDIENTS:

1 cup chopped mango

2 cup Strawberries chopped (set one cup aside)

6 ounces Nonfat vanilla yogurt

1 teaspoon Vanilla extract

2 teaspoons Granulated sugar

1/4 cup Orange juice

1 cup Raspberries (set 1/2 cup aside)

2 tablespoons lemon juice

8 Vanilla wafers

DIRECTIONS:

Combine the mango, 1 cup strawberries, yogurt, vanilla, sugar, and orange juice. Puree in a stationary blender or with an immersion blender until smooth. Fold in the remaining berries. Crush and sprinkle 1 vanilla wafer on each serving.

NUTRITION:

Approximately 8 servings

Calories: 87

Protein: 2 grams

Carbohydrate: 17 grams

Sodium: 45 milligrams

Fat: 1 gram

Fiber: 2 grams

TROPICAL PUNCH PARFAIT

This was my first published recipe. I couldn't resist adding it here.

INGREDIENTS:

1 cup Mango diced (approximately 1 medium)

1 cup Pineapple chunks

2 Tangerines peeled and sectioned

1 medium Banana sliced

1 tablespoon rum extract

1 tablespoon lime juice

1/2 teaspoon nutmeg

2 ounces apricot nectar

1/2 cup nonfat vanilla frozen yogurt or ice cream per serving

DIRECTIONS:

Mix together all of the ingredients except the frozen yogurt. Refrigerate for at least 1 hour. Scoop 1/2 cup frozen yogurt into a parfait or margarita style glass, then top with 1/2 cup of the fruit mixture.

NUTRITION:

Approximately 8 servings

Calories: 158

Protein: 4.2

fat: 0

Carbohydrates: 37 grams

Fiber: 1 gram

Sodium: 53 milligrams

REFERENCES

- Academy of Nutrition and Dietetics, **www.eatright.org**

- American Cancer Society, **www.cancer.org**

- American College of Sports Medicine, **www.acsm.org**

- American Diabetes Association, **www.diabetes.org**

- American Heart Association, **www.heart.org**

- Calorie King, **www.calorieking.com**

- Center for Science in the Public Interest, **www.cspi.net**

- Consumer lab, **www.consumerlab.com**

- Fit Day, **www.fitday.com**

- Gatorade Sports Science Institute, **www.gssiweb.com**

- Harvard School of Public Health, **www.hsph.harvard.edu/nutrionsource**

- National Heart, Lung and Blood Institute, **www.nhlbi.nih.gov**

- President's Council on Fitness and Sports, **www.fitness.gov**

- Seafood Watch, **www.montereybayaquarium.org**

- Spark People, **www.sparkpeople.com**

Proof

20085390R00071

Made in the USA
Charleston, SC
26 June 2013